RESEARCH METHODOLOGY AND DATA ANALYSIS

E-RECORDS INTEGRITY REQUIREMENTS

RESEARCH METHODOLOGY AND DATA ANALYSIS

Additional books and e-books in this series can be found on Nova's website under the Series tab.

RESEARCH METHODOLOGY AND DATA ANALYSIS

E-RECORDS INTEGRITY REQUIREMENTS

ORLANDO LÓPEZ

nova
science publishers
New York

https://doi.org/10.52305/BALY7555

NOTICE TO THE READER

Library of Congress Cataloging-in-Publication Data

ISBN: 978-1-68507-553-8

Published by Nova Science Publishers, Inc. † New York

This book is dedicated to Rafael López, my father.
I'm a continuation of his story and proud to be your son.
The son of a draftsman.

Contents

FOREWORD

Data integrity has always been implicit within global Good Manufacturing Practice regulations. There has also been an attitude within the pharmaceutical industry of "trust us, our people are trained." Since 2005 and the discovery of the data falsification at Able Laboratories due to a whistleblower calling the local FDA field office, the trust between regulators and industry has eroded. It became apparent that the Agency's inspectors had failed to discover the falsification during seven previous inspections as they focused on paper printouts from computerised systems and not electronic records.

Since then, data integrity has become a major issue globally with many more cases of falsification of records or poor data management practices being discovered throughout the world. This has resulted in a sea change in the attitudes of regulatory authorities globally. More stringent inspections, more guidance documents and industry guidance has been published. The focus of these guidance documents is on ensuring electronic records are complete, consistent and accurate as well as trustworthy and reliable.

However, interpreting regulatory guidance can be difficult when faced with conflicting requirements from different sources. For example, backup means the first stage of a disaster recovery business continuity process, unless you are the FDA where backup is defined as archive in the 2018 Data Integrity and Compliance with cGMP guidance for industry.

A data life cycle is an expectation from regulatory authorities, but this needs to be aligned with a computerised system life cycle covering how computerised systems are configured, implemented and validated. This is important as a computerised system can be validated, yet the electronic records can be vulnerable and subject to manipulation and/or deletion. Data vulnerabilities need to be identified and managed for each computerised system, but not all systems and data are equal. The criticality of data and a system depends on the intended use and here is where risk management is so critical to place scarce resources where they are most needed to mitigate data vulnerabilities.

It is important to realize that data integrity (can I trust the data?) is not the only requirement of GMP electronic records. Using the same record set, data quality (can I make a decision?) must not be forgotten. There is no point in having trustworthy data if they are delivered late or in the wrong format. Therefore, both data integrity and data quality must be considered when designing and implementing computerised systems.

One of the themes running through regulatory and industry guidance documents is sometimes the explicit but often the implicit requirement to remove paper from the process and focus on electronic records generated by computerised systems. For example, *hybrid systems are not encouraged* as well as *hybrid systems should be replaced at the earliest opportunity,* is about as close as a regulatory authority can get to saying "don't use hybrid systems."

Therefore, automation of the pharmaceutical industry is essential as it should facilitate the removal of paper records. However, senior management fail to invest in automation to speed processes, enhance regulatory compliance and remove paper. They have a mindset that if a process was acceptable in the last inspection, it will be acceptable in the next one. This is wrong and there is a requirement in both US and EU regulations for companies to keep current.

This book is intended to address these problems and offer suggestions to improve design of automated systems. It is written by an acknowledged expert in the field who is also a prolific writer.

Bob McDowall
Director
R. D. McDowall Ltd
July 2021

PREFACE

All the e-records created during product manufacturing and analysis must maintain their integrity throughout the product's lifecycle.

As a state or condition, e-records integrity measures the validity and fidelity of related data [1].

E-records integrity is required to change information and programs only in a specified and authorized manner. It is a fundamental element of the quality system in any regulatory authority. The regulated user can use E-records with integrity and many other quality-related characteristics [2] to demonstrate the quality and safety of drugs.

E-records must be protected against alteration without proper permission. E-records integrity technological controls are designed into business processes that create and maintain e-records supporting activities regulated by life science requirements.

Based on the Universal Electronic Records Management (ERM) Requirements, Version 2.03 [3] published by the National Archives and Records Administration (NARA), this book presents the bounded characterization of e-records handling systems. The reader will reference requirements that must be agreed upon between the relevant stakeholders [4].

The documentation, analysis, assessment of the risk, tracing, prioritizing, and agreeing on e-records integrity requirements applicable toe-records handling systems are elements of requirements management.

The e-records handling systems must ensure that the e-records a stored, archived or disposed of safely and securely. It includes the e-records integrity information critical to understanding the problem and supporting relevant stakeholders in its resolution.

As in my previous two books written about data integrity [5, 6], out of the scope of this book are the behavioral aspects of regulated life science industries that knowingly employ unreliable or unlawful activities.

Enjoy the reading. If you have any suggestions for improvement or questions, send them to olopez6102@msn.com.

Orlando López
SME – E-records Integrity
Winter 2021-22

References

[1] Data is defined as the contents of a record. It is the basic unit of information with a unique meaning and can be transmitted. (ISO/IEC 17025).

[2] López, O., "Introduction to Data Quality," in *Ensuring the Integrity of Electronic Health Records*, López, O., Ed. (Routledge, Boca Ratón, FL, 1st ed., 2021), pp. 219-228.

[3] https://www.archives.gov/records-mgmt/policy/universalerm requirements

[4] A stakeholder is anyone who has a stake in the project's successful outcome – system owner(s), business managers, regulated end-users, quality assurance, software engineers, support people, and so forth.

[5] López, O., "*Data Integrity in Pharmaceutical and Medical Devices Regulation Operations*," Eds. (CRC Press, Boca Raton, FL, 1st ed., 2017).

[6] López, O., "*Ensuring the Integrity of Electronic Health Records,*" Routledge, Boca Ratón, Fl., 2021.

Chapter 1

INTRODUCTION

It is an expectation by the regulatory authorities that the associated e-records of electronic systems [1] performing regulated activities are not altered accidentally or maliciously by an unauthorized manner. The relevant stakeholders will be catalogued such unauthorized alterations that the system is without the proper data integrity (DI) controls and would be deemed a noticeable deficiency.

As in my previous two books written about data integrity [2, 3], the DI definition I use is originated from the National Institute of Standards and Technology (NIST) [4].

This book covers the requirements applicable to DI in the medicines' manufacturing practices regulations, pharmaceutical and biotechnological. These requirements were taken from the Universal Electronic Records Management (ERM) Requirements, Version 2.03 [5], and published by the National Archives and Records Administration (NARA). Careful editing was necessary to fit the context of this book.

It guides system developers and buyers of systems.

This book is divided into fifteen chapters and six appendices. It is relevant to production systems and quality control systems medicines manufacturers.

Chapter 2, What is data integrity? Defines the concept of DI using the NIST E-records Integrity definition and concepts. It is based on a presentation about the same subject in August 2018 [6].

As information objects, electronic records have a lifecycle. Chapter 3, E-Records Lifecycle, discusses the e-records lifecycle.

Chapter 4, Management of Computer Systems Requirements, re-visits this software engineering significant subject. The success or failure of any project is based on the correct definition and the attributes of requirements.

Chapter 5 describes the integration between computer systems and e-records lifecycles.

Chapter 6 Risk Management addresses the tasks and plans that help avoid risk and help minimize damage.

The ERM DI requirements are addressed in seven chapters, from Chapter 7 to Chapter 13.

Chapter 7, Supporting Services, discusses explicitly the requirements related to the design and implementation of the regulated policies and procedures.

Delineated by the e-records lifecycle, Chapters 8-13 cover the main requirements applicable to DI: Capture, Maintenance and Use, Disposal, Transfer, Metadata, and Reporting. These ERM requirements are translated to the production systems and quality control systems environments that are found in the manufacturers of the medicines.

The vulnerabilities to the e-records may be used to undermine the quality of records and may ultimately undermine the quality of medicinal products [7]. Chapter 14 examines the typical vulnerabilities of e-records and the association of the vulnerabilities with data integrity requirements.

Data integrity refers to whether data is trustworthy. Just because the information is trustworthy does not mean it is also useful. The usefulness of data is achieved by implementing data quality into data handling practices. Elements to consider in data quality are presented in Chapter 15. This chapter aims to modify the mind-frame in our industry and establish data quality in our practices.

It is not the intention of this book to develop a standard for the regulated industry. This book intends to guide how the industry can effectively manage e-records integrity vulnerabilities and raise essential compliance in this area based on standards already written by others.

Except for the definition of DI, this book is consistent with the DI guidelines recently published, especially with the Pharmaceutical Inspection Convention and Pharmaceutical Inspection Co-operation Scheme (PIC/S) [8] and Medicines and Healthcare Products Regulatory Agency (MHRA) [9] DI guidance documents.

As described in this book, the recommendations to implement the e-records controls are purely from the standpoint and opinion of the authors and should serve as a suggestion only. They are not intended to serve as the regulators' official implementation process.

References

[1] *Electronic systems mean systems, including hardware and software, that produce electronic records.*

[2] López, O., "*Data Integrity in Pharmaceutical and Medical Devices Regulation Operations,*" Eds. (CRC Press, Boca Raton, FL, 1st ed., 2017).

[3] López, O., "*Ensuring the Integrity of Electronic Health Records,*" Routledge, Boca Ratón, Fl., 2021.

[4] *Data Integrity - The property that the data is complete and has not been altered in an unauthorized manner.* Data integrity covers data entry or collection, storage, transmission, and processing. (NIST SP 800-57P1)

[5] https://www.archives.gov/records-mgmt/policy/universalermrequirements

[6] López, O., "*Comparison of Health Authorities Data Integrity Expectations,*" paper presented at the IVT 4th Annual Data Integrity Validation, Cambridge, MA, 15-16 August 2018.

[7] Russia Federal State Institute of Drugs and Good Practices, "*Data Integrity & Computer System Validation Guideline,*" September 2018 (Draft).

[8] PIC/S PI-041-3, "*Good Practices for Data Management and Integrity in Regulated GMP/GDP Environments*," (Pharmaceu-tical Inspection Convention/Pharmaceutical Inspection Cooperation Scheme, Geneva, Switzerland, 2021).

[9] MHRA, "*GXP Data Integrity Guidance and Definition,*" (Medicines and Healthcare products Regulatory Agency, London, UK, 2018).

Chapter 2

What Is Data Integrity?

Introduction

A reliable or trustworthy electronic system consists of a computer infrastructure, applications, and procedures that:

- are reasonably suited to performing their intended functions,
- provide a sufficiently reliable level of availability, reliability and correct operation,
- are reasonably secure from intrusion and misuse, and
- adhere to generally accepted security principles.

The objectives of a trustworthy electronic system are to ensure:

- Confidentiality – provides the ability to keep company confidential information private by preventing unauthorized access. It is the state of keeping or being kept secret or private.
- Integrity – offers consistency of data; in particular, preventing unauthorized creation, alteration, or destruction of data and, it ensures that when an authorized person makes a change that should not have been made, can be reversed the damage.

- Availability – legitimate users are not improperly denied access to information and resources.

Confidentiality, integrity, and availability (CIA) is the triad assurance model [1]. CIA triad is considered the three most essential components of security. It highlights core data security objectives and guides organizations to keep their confidential data protected from unauthorized access and data exfiltration [2].

The simple best practices to the CIA triad are:

- Categorize data and assets being handled based on their regulatory criticality.
- Require data encryption and two-factor authentication to be the basic security technique restricting access to the electronic systems to unauthorized regulated users. (EU Annex 11 p 12.1 [3])
- Ensure that access control lists, file permissions and associated lists are monitored and updated regularly. (EU Annex 11 p 12.3 [3])

DATA INTEGRITY

In my first book about data integrity [4], I used the following definition of data integrity as "*the property that data have not been altered in an unauthorized manner while in transit, during processing or in storage*" [5]. In my second book on the same subject [6], I added "*since it was created*" [7]. The definition of data integrity I'm currently using is "*the property that data has not been altered in an unauthorized manner since it was created, in storage, during processing or while in transit.*" Refer to Figure 2.1.

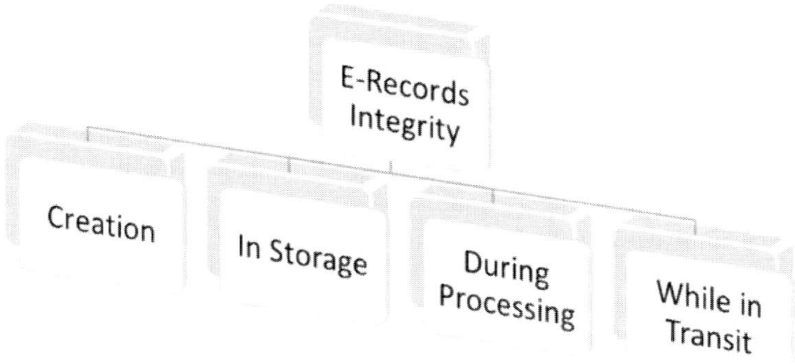

Figure 2.1. E-records Integrity.

Logical controls of the systems must be in place for the network (i.e., local area network (LAN), wide area network (WAN)), for the repository for electronic records (i.e., data server), and within the database (i.e., Oracle). Access to the systems, solutions and electronic documentation may depend on access to the network.

Physical controls are in place to protect the hardware on which the solutions and data servers, where the associated e-records reside.

The appropriate information technology (IT) platform group assigns and grants specific operating system and database access based on recommendations and approval from the system owner.

The e-records integrity is compromised after an unauthorized modification is performed; subsequently, the e-record has been altered or destroyed, inadvertently or accidentally.

Some controls to protect e-records are [8]:

- Provide access to only authorized individuals.
- Access to the data should verify identity in some way. For example, device checks (US FDA 21 CFR Part 11.10(h)) are an example of verifying the validity of the source system where the source data is coming from.
- Use encryption. Scramble and allow the data in a format where the only way can see the data is if a key is provided.

To prevent changes to data in an unauthorized manner:

- Use specialized software that monitors suspicious activities and notify someone of unauthorized modifications to the data.
- Keep systems current and upgrade when necessary.
- The backup system regularly and store the backup in an offsite location.

REFERENCES

[1] https://whatis.techtarget.com/definition/Confidentiality-integrity-and-availability-CIA.

[2] Data exfiltration is sometimes referred to as data extrusion, data exportation, or data theft. All these terms are used to describe the unauthorized transfer of data from a computer or other device. (https://digitalguardian.com/blog/what-data-exfiltration)

[3] Computerized systems. In: *The rules governing medicinal products in the European Union.* Volume 4: Good manufacturing practice (GMP) guidelines: Annex 11, June 2011.

[4] López, O., "*Data Integrity in Pharmaceutical and Medical Devices Regulation Operations: Best Practices Guide to Electronic Records Compliance,*" CRC Press, Boca Ratón, Fl., 2017.

[5] NIST SP 88-33, "*Underlying Technical Models for Information Technology Security,*" December 2001, (Withdrawn: August 2018).

[6] López, O., "*Ensuring the Integrity of Electronic Health Records,*" Routledge, Boca Ratón, Fl., 2021.

[7] NIST SP 800-57, "*Recommendation for Key Management: Part 1 – General,*" May 2020.

[8] US FDA 21 CFR Part 11.10(c).

Additional Readings

The following are the data integrity publications. These can be found at https://drive.google.com/drive/folders/1pB9XE29MuFpCBmNpQq0iG8RubmOCPe-u

CEFIC, "Practical risk-based guide for managing data integrity," March 2019 (Version 1).

Federal State Institute of Drugs and Good Practices (Russian), "Data Integrity & Computer System Validation," (Draft) August 2018.

Health Canada, "Good Manufacturing Practices (GMP) Guidelines," 2018 Edition, Version 3 (GUI-0001).

ICH, "Integrated Addendum to ICH Guideline GCP E6(R1)," November 2016.

IPEC, "Data Integrity for Pharmaceutical Grade Excipients," April 2020.

MHRA, "GXP Data Integrity Guidance and Definition," (Medicines and Healthcare products Regulatory Agency, London, UK, March 2018).

National Medical Products Association (NMPA (former CFDA)), "Drug Data Management Practices Guidance," December 2020.

US FDA, "*Guidance for Industry Data Integrity and Compliance with Drug CGMP Questions and Answers*," (Food and Drug Administration, Silver Spring, Maryland, USA, 2018).

PIC/S PI-041-1 "Good Practices for Data Management and Integrity in Regulated GMP/GDP Environments," (Pharmaceu-tical Inspection Convention/Pharmaceutical Inspection Cooperation Scheme, Geneva, Switzerland, July 2021).

EU OMLC, "Management of documents and records," January 2016 (6R).

OECD, "Advisory Document on GLP Data Integrity," September 2021 (Final).

WHO, "*Guideline on Data Integrity*" (QAS/19.819 Draft), October 2019.

Chapter 3

E-RECORDS LIFECYCLE [1]

INTRODUCTION

Electronic records [2] (e-records) have a lifecycle as information objects. The e-records lifecycle refers to the following electronic systems activities [3]:

- Capture and creation of data.
- Processing into usable information
- Checking the completeness and accuracy of reported data and processed information.
- E-records are used to make a decision.
- Inactive Phase by retaining and retrieval of data which protects it from loss or unauthorized amendment.
- Final disposition by retiring data in a controlled manner at the end of its life.

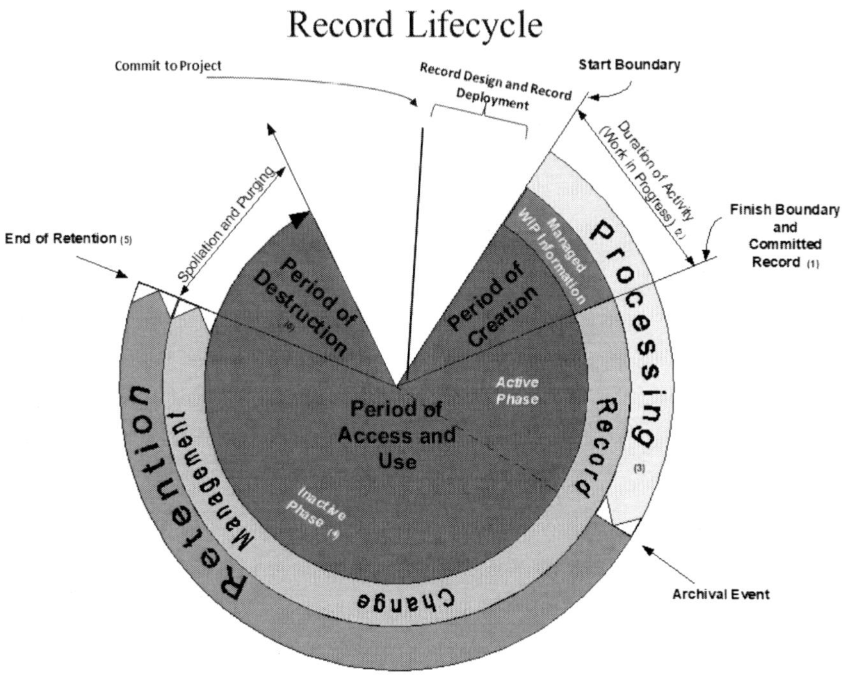

Figure 3.1. E-records Lifecycle.

In my previous book [4] the e-records lifecycle's phases, Figure 3.1, are Data Process Design, Data Capture, E-records Creation, Active E-records, Inactive E-records, and E-records Final Disposition.

Because this book it is discussed the Universal ERM Requirements (Version 2.03, and published by NARA, the e-records lifecycle phases are the same ones contained in the ERM Requirements: Capture, Maintenance and Use Disposal, and Transfer.

The correlation of these two e-record lifecycles is:

E-records Lifecycle Phase	Ensuring the Integrity of Electronic Health Records	NARA Universal ERM Requirements -V2.03
1	Data Process Design	
2	Data Capture	Capture
3	E-records Creation	
4	Active E-records	Maintenance and Use
5	Inactive E-records	
6	E-records Final Disposition	Transfer

During the data flow through the system, the e-records integrity can be impacted at any phase in the e-records lifecycle. Consequently, it is vital to assess the data [5] risk and data criticality at all phases [6] to ensure the e-records during the lifecycle.

A risk management approach [7] to data integrity can achieve by considering data risk and criticality at each phase of the e-records lifecycle. The effort applied to assess and implement the control measures should be commensurate with this e-records risk and criticality assessments.

Data Process Design [8]

Records Identification Phase

The Records Identification Phase of the e-records lifecycle is known as strategic e-records planning. Strategic e-records planning determines the information requirements of the operations necessary to collect the e-records and implements a technology-independent set of techniques to arrive at a set of e-records and activity models that represent the current Good Manufacturing Practices (CGMP) process.

Current systems are analyzed for input, output, and operations (forms, reports, and code) to assess the feasibility of reverse engineering or re-engineering.

The e-records models were constructed to form a foundation for developing and defining standard e-records elements. Thus, strategic e-records planning provides a framework where e-records become separate from their processes and constitute a resource independent of applications for e-records use planning.

The strategic e-records planning is based upon the e-records requirements of specific functional processes performed in support of CGMP activities. Strategic e-records planning identifies the e-records required to satisfy particular information requirements most efficiently.

E-records needs also can be identified through fewer formal means such as system change requests.

Records Standardization Phase

During the Records Standardization Phase, the information requirements identified through strategic e-records planning are given common or standard representations. Data profiling is the technical analysis of data to describe its content, consistency, and structure.

The Record Standardization Phase of the e-records lifecycle also addresses actual e-records values (items). There are many instances where the format and attributes of the e-records values must be standardized to ensure consistency across the regulated site/corporate. When e-records must be shared by more than one functional activity, the standardization of e-records values is essential.

The strategic e-records planning establishes common e-records values and provides the framework for standard e-records use. The lines between standardization, acquisition, and maintenance stages become unclear in this area. Once an information requirement is identified and the e-records elements representing that information requirement are defined, the e-records element domains may vary depending on usage.

The established standards will apply to information such as the authority for a specific instance of metadata, the preferred acquisition method and source for populating a database with a particular e-records element, the e-records set owner responsible for the accuracy and/or integrity of the actual e-records values, and numerous other pieces of information. It is helpful to view metadata as a type of controlling framework that outlines a broad set of rules to which the e-records of interest to an enterprise must be complying. The e-records administrator is the caretaker of this framework and its interface with the regulated entity overall mission. The components e-records administrator performs the same functions within their Components for their Component-level strategic e-records planning.

The final product of the Standardization Phase is the approved standard e-records and metadata, including e-records entities, attributes, definitions, and values.

The outcome of the Standardization Phase is employed to create the data flows or linage to connect the data warehouses. Mapping the fields is essential to ensure that during the direct move, each valid e-record from the source is loaded to the appropriate target table(s), connecting precisely two databases.

Capture

The capture of data objects indicates that the data is generated by:

- instrumentation/equipment. The data object is captured by an electronic system [9] (e.g., I/O card as in Figure 3.2).
- an electronic system. The data object is captured the same electronic system (e.g., Big Data integration).
- another computer via a wired/wireless interface. The receiving system captures the data object.
- manually entered by an operator/user (e.g., Supervisory System as in Figure 3.2).

In a typical environment for electronic systems performing activities covered by the medicines' manufacturing practices regulations, Figure 3.2, the data is imported directly from manufacturing equipment or control signals. Data can be entered, as well, manually using the Supervisory System.

The data objects are not necessarily moved from the source system. This only happens in Big Data environments. The Extract Transform Load (ETL) is an integration tool for managing real-time data integration. The target for ETL technology is a database such as a source system, a data warehouse (DW) or data marts (DM).

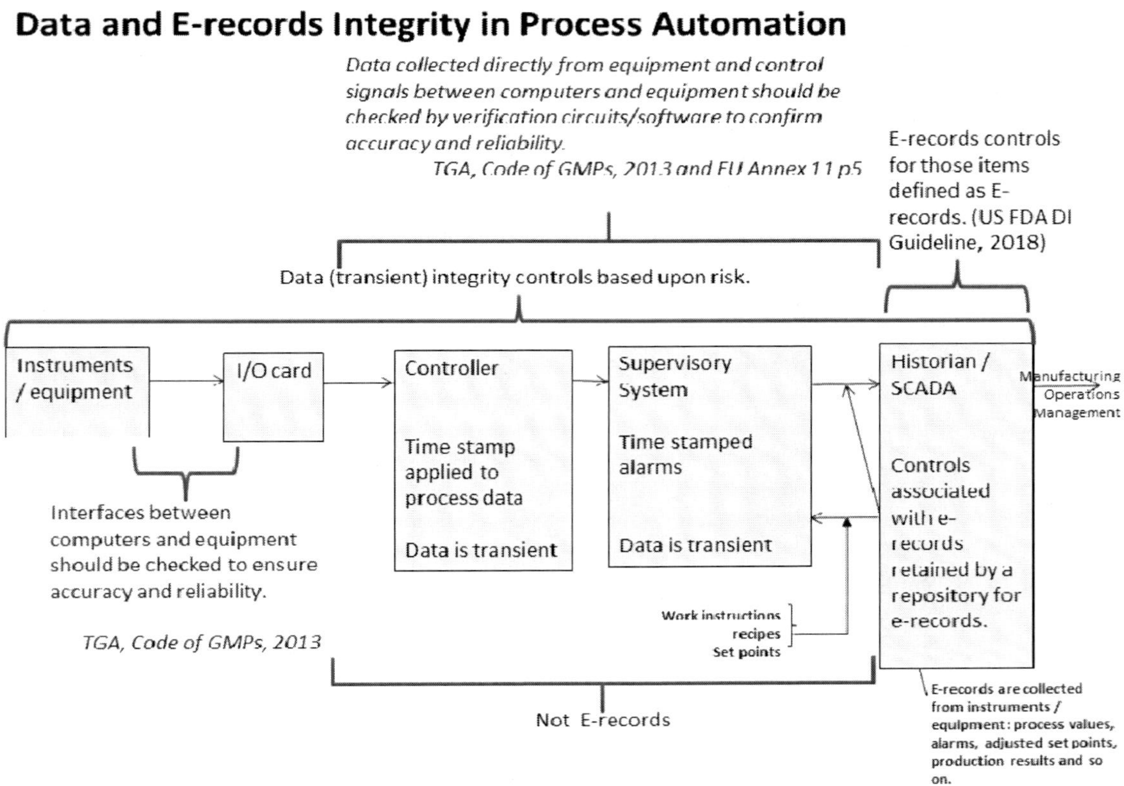

Figure 3.2. Data and E-records Integrity in Process Automation.

Figure 3.2 shows that the data is loaded into the I/O card from the instrument/equipment. The loaded to the controller and supervisory system resides in transient memory. This memory must have a constant power supply or lose the loaded data. The loaded data resident in transient memory is also called transient or temporary data.

In the context of Figure 3.2, the data between the equipment and the electronic storage device (e.g., Supervisory Control and Data Acquisition (SCADA)/Historian) is regarded as transient data.

During the period of 'temporary data' between the equipment and the electronic storage device, there is often limited audit trail provision amending, deleting or manipulating data. Temporary data is a data integrity risk [10].

Removing the use of temporary memory (or reducing the period that data is stored in temporary memory) reduces the risk of undetected data manipulation. Electronic systems should be designed to require saving data contemporaneously [11] to the electronic storage device before prompting users to make changes. If data is not saved contemporaneously, the data must be protected against editing by reasonable means or reprocessed by the human user.

After the data is transformed and the corresponding built-in checks performed, there is a commitment to use the data. The captured data is then created.

CREATION

All transient data become an e-record after the transient data is saved in an electronic repository for e-records [12]. When the transient data is generated to satisfy a CGMP requirement and saved in electronic storage for e-records, the transient data becomes a CGMP e-record [13].

The e-records that are original records retained in the format or processing environment they were originally generated are considered raw data [14].

In Figure 3.2, subsequently, the transient data is written to an electronic repository for e-records as part of the SCADA. The transient data becomes raw data.

The transient data is stored in defined fields, becoming raw data (e.g., structured data). The raw data is used for their intended purposes as representing the activities they stand for. From the time it is saved in an electronic storage device, it can edit the raw data to final disposition.

E-records may include the raw data which is used to generate other records. For e-records, regulated users should define which data are to be used as raw data. At least, all data on which quality decisions are based should be defined as raw data [15].

After the transient data becomes raw data and, at the same time, e-record, the designed physical and logical controls to the e-records must be in place using the data handling function. These controls include physical protections, stamped audit trail, records handling [16], archival and retrieval. In Figure 3.2, the alarms and the associated actions to the alarms actions taken at the Supervisory System are managed by the programmable logic controller (PLC). The associated alarm records are saved in the corresponding electronic repository system at the storage device level.

To recap, creation is the process of placing an object data under e-records management control for disposition and access purposes. E-records can be imported from other sources or manually entered into the system.

Must be created the correct records to meet the needs of business policy, governmental regulations, and legal purposes. They must be correctly and reliably reflecting or representing the associate action, activity, or event. The correct records require that they are created in an environment that ensures authenticity and integrity [3].

ACTIVE

During the Active Phase, data interacts with other pieces of information, is transformed, and is utilized in various reports.

The Active Phase of an e-record encompasses e-records that are kept and accessed from the processing environment for their intended purpose. Activities associated are the store, use, processes (transforming and migrating), modifications, periodically reviewing, analyzing, reporting, retaining, backing up, and restoring. This includes ensuring records are migrated and converted as systems change, so the records remain usable.

In addition to the audit trail functionality during this phase, change management may represent governance that controls editing or modifying the e-records.

The criticality of the raw data, periodically, may cleanse raw data within the e-records to correct inconsistent values after using the data. This activity must be suitably managed using procedural control and must be documented (e.g., audit trail).

The three essential CGMP controls to e-records in storage compliant with e-records integrity are:

- the modifications to CGMP e-records must be recorded at the time of the modification, including the audit trail.
- Periodic backups must be performed.
- must establish security controls for all e-records storages as a means of ensuring e-records protections.

The process of managing records through their most active phase includes ensuring records are migrated and transformed as systems change, so the records remain usable.

Inactive and Final Disposition

Inactive Phase

E-records that are inactive, superseded, replaced, or withdrawn are inactivated. The e-records in scope are ingested [17].

When acquiring or developing the electronic archive, it is expected consideration must be given to the long-term retention schedule requirements for these e-records, particularly concerning accessibility, readability, traceability and possibly any future processing needs through to final disposition.

Technical and functional requirement specifications for such electronic archives should include long-term storage, preservation, management and retrieval of their e-records. The requirements should include all the issues described in this section to ensure that e-records from these electronic archives can be archived in a manner compliant with all applicable requirements and industry best practices.

The key activities associated with maintaining inactive e-records are store, access, periodically reviewing, reporting, transferring, retaining, backing up, and restoring.

Three essential requirements to maintain inactive CGMP e-records are:

- the archiving process must include verification that all e-records and associated metadata are not altered in value and/or meaning during the migration process.
- archived e-records need to be verified periodically for accessibility, readability, integrity, and the state of security.
- periodic backups must be performed.

Final Disposition

The primary tool used to manage the final disposition of e-records is the e-records schedule. An e-records plan is an official e-records and information retention and disposal policy. The schedule provides mandatory instructions for keeping records and no record materials that are no longer needed for current business.

After meeting the approved retention time, the e-records are scheduled for destruction and physically erased according to an approved procedure. The Final Disposition Phase is noticeably short and includes discarding content, metadata, audit trails, documentation, and any pointers to the e-record and connections to related records.

As part of a regulated entity's records handling program, the current good practice also includes a periodic practice to revisit the approved retention of periods of specific records as business, regulatory or legal requirements change. From a legal perspective, it is important to consider that e-record handling programs include defined provisions to suspend the execution of the purge process (including backup tapes) when records are part of a legal discovery process during pending litigation.

Purging e-records and paper records are the last steps in the record lifecycle. Must follow it the reliable execution of the purging procedural control for the deletion of CGMP e-records [18].

METADATA

Metadata are elements of information that answer the questions 'who, what, where, when, and why' regarding electronic records. Metadata elements provide administrative, descriptive, and technical information that describe the structure and content of electronic records. Metadata elements also provide contextual information that explains how e-records were created, used, managed, and maintained before their disposal and how they are related to other records.

Report Generators

The generation of reports allows for further analysis and demonstrate adequate controls and compliance. Reports may include search results, records eligible for disposition, audit logs, and other customized or ad hoc reports.

Principle

Throughout the data lifecycle, records management principles [19] should adhere to the true, accurate, timely data management principles that can be traced back to ensure the reliability of the e-records [20].

References

[1] López, O., "*E-records Lifecycle*," Journal of GXP Compliance, Vol. 19, Issue 4, Nov 2015.

[2] Record – Collection of related data treated as a unit. (ISPE/PDA, "*Technical Report: Good Electronic Records Management* (GERM)," July 2002).

[3] ISPE/PDA, "*Good Practice and Compliance for Electronic Records and Signatures. Part 1 Good Electronic Records Management (GERM).*" July 2002.

[4] López, O., "*Ensuring the Integrity of Electronic Health Records*," Routledge, Boca Ratón, Fl., 2021.

[5] Data – data is defined as the contents of a record. It is the basic unit of information with a unique meaning and can be transmitted (ISO/IEC 17025).

[6] EU, "*Questions and Answers: Good Manufacturing Practice and Good Distribution Practice, Data Integrity*," August 2016, https://www.ema.europa.eu/en/human-regulatory/research-

development/compliance/good-manufacturing-practice/guidance-good-manufacturing-practice-good-distribution-practice-questions-answers#data-integrity-(new-august-2016)-section

[7] ICH, *Q9 Quality Risk Management*, November 2005.

[8] López, O., "Introduction to Data Quality," *Journal of Validation Technology*, Vol 26 Issue 2, April 2020.

[9] *Electronic systems - Systems, including hardware and software, that produce electronic records.*

[10] EU, "*Questions and Answers: Good Manufacturing Practice and Good Distribution Practice, Data Integrity*," August 2016.

[11] Contemporaneous - The evidence of actions, events or decisions should be recorded as they take place. (PIC/S PI 041-1, "*Good Practice for Data Management and Integrity in Regulated GMP GDP Environments*," July 2021).

[12] Repository of e-records - A direct access device on which the electronic records and metadata are stored.

[13] US FDA, "*Guidance for Industry Data Integrity and Compliance with Drug CGMP Questions and Answers*," (Food and Drug Administration, Silver Spring, Maryland, USA, December 2018).

[14] Raw Data - Original records and documentation, retained in the format in which they were originally recorded (i.e., paper or electronic), or as a 'true copy.'

[15] *EudraLex*, Volume 4 Good Manufacturing Practice (GMP) Guidelines, Chapter 4 Documentation (European Commission, Brussels, Belgium, 2011. 4).

[16] Data Handling - The process of ensuring that data is stored, archived, or disposed of safely and securely during the data lifecycle.

[17] Ingestion - The process that accepts e-records for archiving.

[18] ECA, "*Deletion of Data: Does it have to be regulated in an SOP?*" June 2019, https://www.gmp-compliance.org/gmp-news/deletion-of-data-does-it-have-to-be-regulated-in-a-sop

[19] Record Management - The planning, controlling, directing, organizing, training, promoting, and other managerial activities

involving the lifecycle of information, including creation, maintenance (use, storage, retrieval), and disposal, regardless of media. Record management procedures are used to achieve adequate and proper documentation of Federal policies and transactions and effective and economic management of Agency/organizational operations. (44 U.S.C. 2901)

[20] NMPA (former CFDA), "*Drug Data Management Practices Guidance*," December 2020.

Additional Reading

UK Government, "*The Data Lifecycle*," in the Government Data Quality Framework, https://www.gov.uk/government/publications/the-government-data-quality-framework/the-government-data-quality-framework#The-Data-Lifecycle

Chapter 4

MANAGEMENT OF COMPUTER SYSTEM REQUIREMENTS [1]

INTRODUCTION

A requirement is a need or expectation that is stated, generally implied or obligatory. "Generally implied" means that it is common practice for the relevant stakeholder such that its absence would be deemed an obvious shortcoming.

The term "requirement" defines a bounded characterization of the system scope that different relevant stakeholders can generate. It includes the information essential to communicate an understanding of the problem and to support relevant stakeholders in its resolution. Various requirements include product, functionality, performance, regulatory, legal, reliability, supportability, usability, security, and non-functional requirements.

Most computer system failures are due to poor requirements gathering and management. It includes not understanding the business impact, what the customer wants, and how the stakeholder interacts with the computer system. This situation negatively affects subsequent development activities, associated work products, and quality.

Requirements management is the process of documenting, analyzing, assessing the risk, tracing, prioritizing, and agreeing on requirements and then controlling change and communicating to relevant stakeholders [2]. It is a continuous process throughout a project.

According to the American Society for Testing and Materials (ASTM) E2500-13 [3], requirements come from four areas: product knowledge, process knowledge, regulatory agencies, and company quality standards.

Requirements may be captured as user scenarios, function and feature lists, analysis models or specifications. These work products are used as a framework to select the supplier/integrator, develop other work products associated with the computer system's development, develop the user acceptance plan/test, and develop the maintenance/operational procedural controls.

Requirement's engineering strives to understand what the relevant stakeholders need and want before designing and building a solution. Tools that software engineers can leverage include Six Sigma, voice of the customer (VOC), quality function deployment (QFD), failure mode and effect analysis (FMEA), requirements analysis matrix (RAM), orthogonal array (OA), cause and effect Analyses (C-E), design structure matrix (DSM), Pugh matrix, and so on.

The requirements engineering tasks comprise:

- Inception - is used context-free questions to establish a basic understanding of the problem, the perspectives of relevant stakeholders who want a solution, the nature of the solution, and the effectiveness of the collaboration between the relevant stakeholders and developers.
- Elicitation – it is found out from the relevant stakeholders what the product objectives are, what is to be done, how the product fits into business needs, and how the product is used daily.
- Elaboration - is developed a refined technical model of software function, behaviour, and information.
- Negotiation - requirements are categorized and organized into subsets, identified requirements, reviewed for correctness, and prioritized based on the relevant stakeholders' needs.

- Specification – requirements are derived from or provided by the relevant stakeholders describing a computer system's function, performance, and development constraints. These work products should be suitable for requirements management through the lifecycle and beyond.
- Requirement's validation - formal technical reviews used to examine the specification work products to ensure requirement quality and that all work products conform to agree upon standards for the process, project, and products.
- Requirements management – activities that help a project team identify, control, and track requirements and requirement changes as the project proceeds.

Figure 4.1 [4] depicts a typical systems development distribution showing the percentage of effort needed for each critical developmental activity. Except for requirements management, front end" activities, including requirements engineering, should take between 40-50% system development lifecycle (SDLC) distribution.

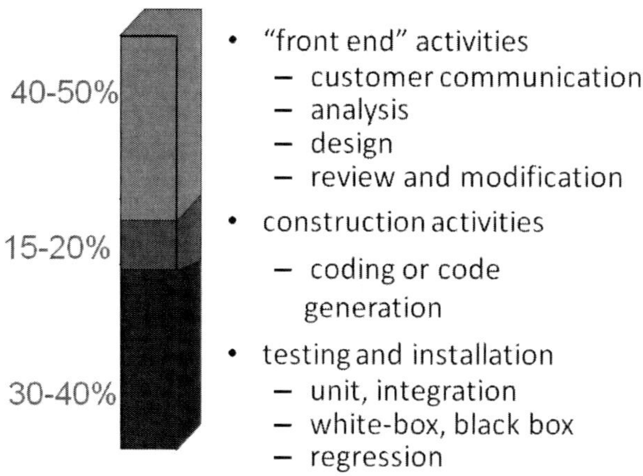

Figure 4.1. Systems Development Distribution.

Figure 4.2 [5] depicts the importance of managing requirements. This figure correlates the cost to find and fix defects during the system lifecycle (SLC). For example, in 1976, the cost to fix an error found after product release was up to 30 times more than one identified in the Design Phase.

This chapter covers the product requirements [6] activities only. Project requirements are out of the scope of this chapter.

REQUIREMENTS MANAGEMENT

The purpose of the Requirements Management process is to maintain and control a current, correct, and documented common understanding of the relevant stakeholders, intended product use, development resources, constraints, and needed computer system capabilities that were captured and baseline in the requirements documentation. It describes the tasks necessary to correct, update, and control a Requirements Specification (RS) [7] document. Figure xx depicts the critical inputs to the RS. Figure 4.2 illustrates the key information to the requirements specification.

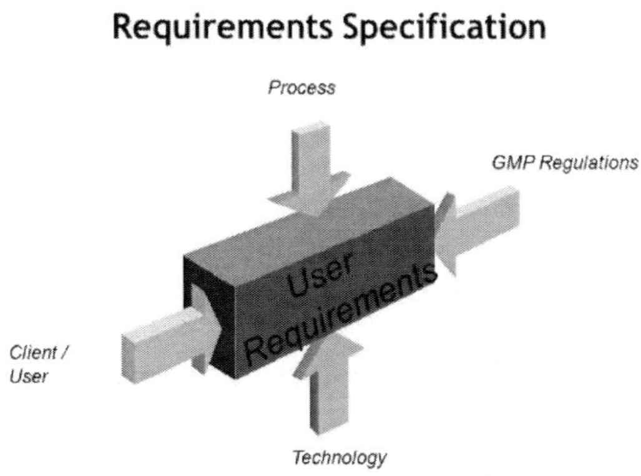

Figure 4.2. Inputs to the Requirements Specification.

The result of the requirements management process is an updated, organized set of documented requirements throughout the system lifecycle that:

- Supports the relevant stakeholder's needs, goals, and objectives.
- Remains within a well-defined scope.

- Identifies and quantifies impacts of changes, including those of scope, schedule, cost, hardware, and staffing.
- Controls the current, documented RS.

A Requirement Management plan may be necessary for highly complex and critical projects. The Requirements Management plan is used to record the activities required to effectively establish [8] the project requirements from the definition, through traceability, to delivery.

The Requirements Management Plan is created during the early Development Period of the SLC (Refer to Chapter 5). Its intended audience is the project manager, project team, project sponsor, and senior leaders whose support is needed to carry out the plan.

According to the Capability, Maturity Model Integration (CMMI) [9], activities as part of the requirements management and can be elements of the plan are:

- Obtaining an Understanding of Requirements.
- Obtaining Commitment to Requirements.
- Managing Requirements Changes.
- Maintaining Bidirectional Traceability of Requirements.
- Ensuring Alignment between Project Work and Requirements.

Requirements Management

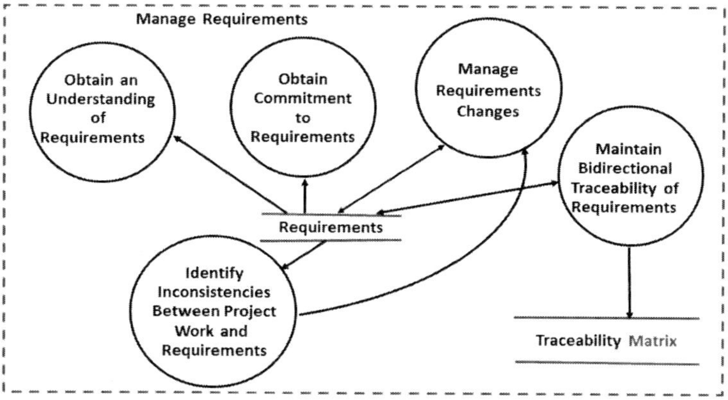

Figure 4.3. Requirements Management.

Figure 4.3 provides the relationships between these activities.

OBTAINING AN UNDERSTANDING OF REQUIREMENTS

The intent is to establish project criteria to identify providers of appropriate requirements, standards for the evaluation and acceptance of requirements, and ensure that the established criteria are met through an analysis or review process.

Those who receive requirements, analyze them with the sources to ensure that a compatible, shared understanding is reached on the meaning of requirements. The result of these analyses and dialogues is an approved RS, including the definition of the system boundaries.

The Quality System regulation requires addressing incomplete, ambiguous, or conflicting requirements. Each requirement (e.g., hardware, software, user, operator interface, and safety) identified in the software requirements specification should be evaluated for accuracy, completeness, consistency, testability, correctness, and clarity. **US FDA 21 CFR 820.30(c).**

Sidebar 4.1. Regulatory Guideline.

Example work products for this practice include:

- Lists of criteria for distinguishing appropriate requirements providers.
- Criteria for evaluation and acceptance of requirements, refer to Table 1.
- Results of analyses against criteria.

Lack of evaluation and acceptance criteria often results in inadequate verification, costly rework or customer rejection.

OBTAINING COMMITMENT TO REQUIREMENTS

Once the understanding of the requirements is established, this practice deals with agreements and commitments among those who have to carry out the activities necessary to implement these requirements.

After getting the commitment of the relevant stakeholders, the main deliverable is the RS. It is an approved document by all relevant stakeholders. The RS establishes the relevant stakeholders' requirements baseline and retains changes of need and their origin throughout the system lifecycle. It is the basis for traceability to the computer system requirements and forms the definitive source of information about requirements for subsequent systems and communications with stakeholders.

Later, the RS will be critical in preventing scope creep or other unnecessary changes in the thick of development. As the system evolves, each new feature opens a world of new possibilities, so the RS anchors the team to the original vision and permits a controlled discussion of scope change.

While many organizations use only documents to manage requirements, others work their requirements baselines using software tools. These tools allow requirements to be managed in a database, and usually have functions to automate traceability (e.g., by allowing electronic links to be created between parent and child requirements, or between test cases and requirements), electronic baseline creation, version control, and change management. Usually, such tools contain an export function that allows a specification document to be created by exporting the requirements data into a standard document application.

The RS must include an overview of the process to familiarize the infrastructure and application developers with the regulated user, business process, regulatory, and data acquisition requirements of the system, and any special considerations for the project. The system functionality must be well defined at the outset to provide the prospective supplier/integrator with enough information to provide a detailed and meaningful proposal. Specifically, the RS must include data definitions; data usage information; data storage, retention, and security requirements; and operational requirements and constraints.

The RS addresses:

- the scope of the system and strategic objectives.
- process overview, sequencing requirements, operational checks.
- sufficient information to enable the supplier/integrator to work on a solution to the problem (e.g., device-driven sequencing, the methods required of the presentation of data, data security, data backup, data and status reporting and trending, and so on).
- redundancy and error-detection protocol.
- operating environment.
- interfaces (e.g., to field devices, data acquisition systems, reports and HMI), I/O lists, communications protocols and data link requirements.
- the information gained from operators and supervisors on the system design requirements and expectations to influence how the system is designed and operated.
- type of control and process operations to be performed.
- data storage requirements.
- transaction/data timing requirements and considerations.
- regulatory requirements.
- preliminary evaluation of the technology.
- feasibility study and preliminary risk assessment.
- safety and security considerations.
- security, other requirements.
- non-functional requirements (e.g., SLC development standards, programming language standards, program naming convention standards, etc.).

Each requirement in the RS should have the attributes depicted in Table 1.

The requirements should be verified during each phase of the SDLC. In a classic "V" model, the requirements are tested during the user acceptance testing, aka the performance qualification (PQ) in the US FDA regulated industries context. This testing should include verifying the procedural controls associated with the system identified in the RS.

MANAGING REQUIREMENTS CHANGES

Once commitments to the requirements are established and plans have been made, the project will transform from planning mode to execution mode. During the project execution phase, possible conditions precipitating a change are:

- A new requirement is identified.
- The software project is re-scoped (requirements added, dropped or modified).
- An inconsistency is identified between the capabilities of the developed product and the documented requirements.

Figure 4.4 depicts that inputs and outputs of the management of requirements changes.

Table 1. Attributes of requirements

Attribute	Definition
Unambiguous	All requirements must have only one interpretation. • Clearly and properly stated. • Complete.
Verifiable	A human being or a machine must be able to verify that the system correctly enacts the stated requirements.
Traceable	The requirements must be traceable from other design and test documents. To facilitate traceability, each requirement should be uniquely identified.
Modifiable	Unanticipated changes must be able to be made easily.
Usable	Each requirement must be tied to business values, identified as a priority for the customer, and appropriately implemented by the development team. The RS must be usable by the development team and subsequent maintenance teams who will be called upon to modify and change the system.
Consistent	Individual requirements must not conflict with each other. Requirements must be consistent with the overall architectural approach and quality attribute priorities.
Complete	It must contain explicit descriptions of all features and functions of the system. It must incorporate definitions of all known situations the system could encounter

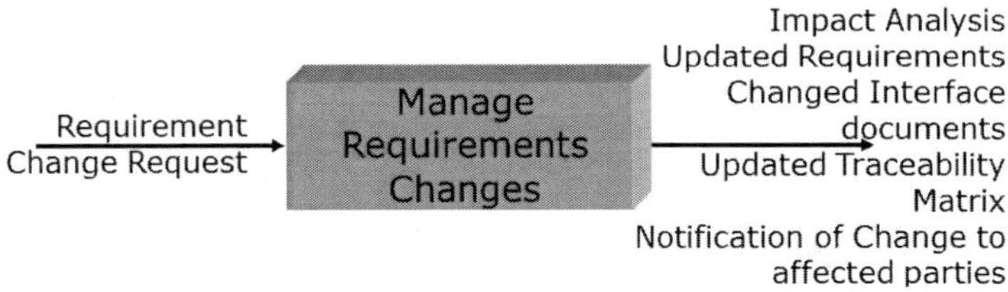

Figure 4.4. Management Requirements Changes.

The entry criterion to this process is:

- A Requirement Change Request has been submitted.

The tasks associated with this process include:

- Analyze change requests for impact and feasibility.
- Prepare an impact analysis statement.
- Determine the disposition of the change request (e.g., accept, reject, defer)

If the change request is accepted, then:

- Generate changed RS, and change requests for other controlled products as applicable and necessary.
- Implement the change. Also, make the necessary modifications to related artefacts: RS, modelling diagrams, QFD, generic specifications, and so on.
- Verify and Validate changed RS.
- Update and distribute updated documentation as necessary.

The exit criteria to this process are:

- A decision was made through the application process not to proceed with the change.
- Updates to requirements made, distributed and controlled.
- Other work product change requests have been generated as required.

As part of the Manage Requirement Changes, the impact analysis process by itself has multiple steps. This process must be clearly defined and communicated to the customer and the project team. The high-level steps of the change impact analysis process include:

1. Get a changed request.
2. Expand the demand statement using Voice of the Customer (VOC) analysis (who, what, when, where, why, and how)
3. Analyze engineering impacts
   a. The "how's" yield clues around impacted features
   b. Identify, for example, quality function deployment (QFD), associated functionality and design parameters. These design parameters are the engineering items to be scrutinized to determine their impact.
4. In review meeting(s) analyze if a problem requires only a hardware/machine "tweak" or if it requires a software change
5. Analyze software impacts.
   a. Using the QFD, identify all the functionalities (use cases) that are impacted.
   b. For each use case, analyze the traceability analysis and the graphical user interface (GUI) and controller change required.
   c. Conduct risk analysis, for example, based on failure mode and effect analysis (FMEA), so the potential regressive damage due to the change is minimized.
6. Create the change request impact analysis document and review it with the customer.

Maintaining Bidirectional Traceability of Requirements

Requirement's traceability (Figure 4.5) is concerned with documenting the origin of a requirement and the relationships between requirements and other development artefacts, such as designs, models, analysis results, code and test plans/cases/procedures/results.

A software requirements traceability analysis should be conducted to trace software requirements to (and from) system requirements and to risk analysis results

Sidebar 4.2. US FDA General Principles of Software Validation.

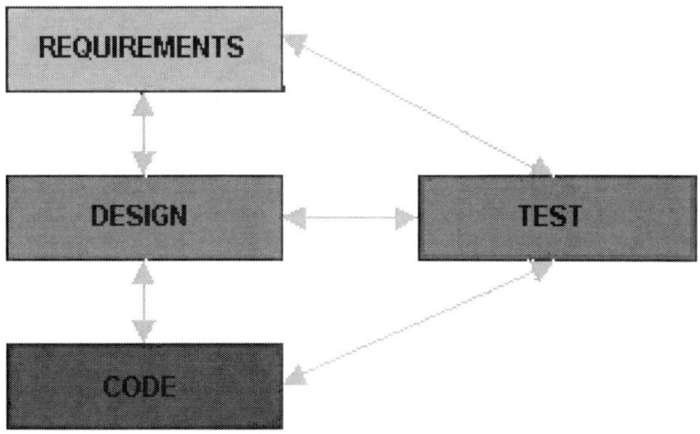

Figure 4.5. Requirements Traceability.

The purpose of requirements traceability is to facilitate:

- overall quality.
- understanding of the product.
- tests necessary to verify.
- ability to manage change.

This practice intends to maintain the bidirectional traceability of requirements for each level of product decomposition. Refer to Figure 4.6.

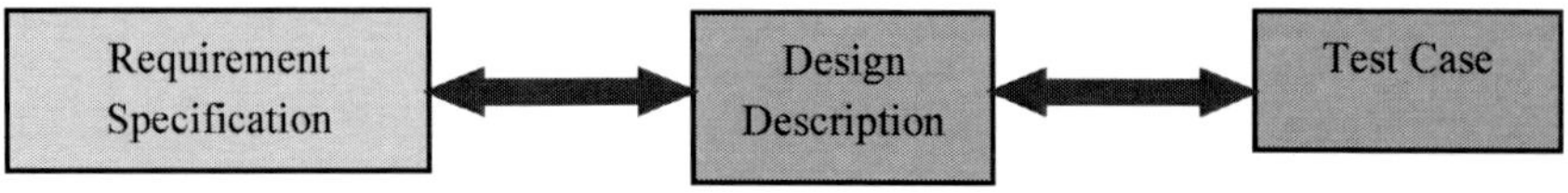

Figure 4.6. Forward/Backward Traceability.

The following two types of traceability are recommended:

1. Forward traceability (i.e., to all documents spawned by the SRS). This depends upon each requirement in the SRS having a unique name or reference number.
2. Backward traceability (i.e., to previous stages of development). This depends upon each requirement explicitly referencing its source in earlier documents.

The forward traceability of the RS is essential when the software product enters the operation and maintenance phase. As code and design documents are modified, it is essential to ascertain the complete set of requirements that may be affected by those modifications.

It should be possible to trace back to the origin of each requirement, and every change made to the requirement should therefore be documented to achieve traceability.

Requirement's traceability is also useful when conducting impact assessments of changes to requirements, design or other configured items.

When the requirements are managed well, they can establish traceability from the source requirement to its lower-level requirements and from the lower-level requirements back to their source. Such bidirectional traceability helps determine that all source requirements have been completely addressed and that all lower-level requirements can be traced to a valid source.

The example below shows the links that are to be maintained. To demonstrate bi-directional traceability, each column's evidence of sorting (and use) is to be captured.

Unique Requirement ID	Requirement Description	Design Reference	Module/Configured Item Reference	Release Reference	Test Script Name/Step Number Reference

Table 2. Traceability activities and SLC

SLC Phase	Typical Traceability Task(s)	Comment
Requirements	• Software Requirements to System Requirements (and vice versa) • Software Requirements to Risk Analysis	A traceability analysis should be conducted to verify that the software design implements all software requirements. As a technique for identifying where requirements are insufficient, the traceability analysis should also verify that all aspects of the design are traceable to software requirements.
Design	• Design Specification to Software Requirements (and vice versa)	It should conduct a traceability analysis to verify that the software design implements all the software requirements. As a technique for identifying where requirements are insufficient, the traceability analysis should also verify that all aspects of the design are traceable to software requirements. Communication links should be analyzed to evaluate the proposed design concerning hardware, user, and related software requirements.
Construction/Source Code/Configuration	• Source Code to Design Specification (and vice versa) • Test Cases to Source Code and Design Specification	A source code traceability analysis is essential to verify that all code is linked to established specifications and test procedures. A source code traceability analysis should be conducted and documented to demonstrate that: • Each element of the software design specification has been implemented in code. • Modules and functions implemented in code can be traced back to an element in the software design specification and the risk analysis. • Tests for modules and functions can be traced back to an element in the software design specification and the risk analysis; and • Tests for modules and functions can be traced to source code for the same modules and functions.
Developer's Software Testing	• Unit (Module) Tests to Detailed Design • Integration Tests to High-Level Design • System Tests to System Requirements	Control measures, such as a traceability analysis, should be used to ensure that the intended coverage is achieved.

Table 2. Continued.

SLC Phase	Typical Traceability Task(s)	• Comment
User Acceptance Testing	User Acceptance Test to System Requirements	• In a typical "V" model, this is the ultimate test. Each requirement must map to at least one test case. • Control measures, such as a traceability analysis, should be used to ensure that the intended coverage is achieved.
Maintenance		After the computer system has been delivered for operations, the forward traceability of the RS is essential when the software product enters the maintenance phase. As part of the activities to conclude a project, the Requirements Traceability Matrix must be updated with the as-built information. The objective is to have an up-to-date matrix describing how the final system design satisfied the requirements document's functional, business, security, and technical specifications. As code and design documents are modified, it is essential to be able to ascertain the complete set of requirements that may be affected by those modifications. A new cycle begins with the new project to the requirements management process.

Traceability is an essential aspect during the verification activities in the SLC, and it is an essential input into design reviews. A formal design review is recommended to confirm that requirements are fully specified and appropriate before extensive software design efforts begin.

Table 2 depicts the traceability activities during a typical SLC.

The practice of requirements traceability is iterative. It is conducted throughout the SLC and involves the following activities:

- Functionality – defining functional requirements based on technical assumptions and/or client needs.
- Traceability – setting up and maintaining a requirements traceability system.

- Log - updating the traceability matrix regularly (at least weekly) with new information.
- Communicating – communicating regularly (at least weekly) with stakeholders about the status of requirements.
- Log – recording data used to track the requirements in the traceability matrix.
- Communication – communicating to stakeholders that a particular requirement has been completed.

The traceability of requirements can be built into documentation and code without having to have a separate traceability document. Three common approaches are traceability matrix, using computer databases to evaluate traceability, and building inherent traceability into the documentation and code structure. Software developers have flexibility in how they want to implement traceability.

ENSURING ALIGNMENT BETWEEN PROJECT WORK AND REQUIREMENTS

This practice focuses on maintaining consistency between requirements, project plans, work products and, in case of inconsistencies, initiates corrective actions to resolve them. For example, should revise the project plan if changes to the requirements are identified as impacting the schedule.

Corrective actions taken by the project to resolve inconsistencies can also result in changes to project plans and supplier agreements.

SUMMARY

It is necessary to identify, control, and track requirements before the design and construction of a computer system can begin.

The Requirements Management consists of five activities:

- Obtaining an Understanding of Requirements.
- Obtaining Commitment to Requirements.
- Managing Requirements Changes.
- Maintaining Bidirectional Traceability of Requirements.
- Ensuring Alignment Between Project Work and Requirements.

The relevance of the Requirements Management to successfully manage a computer system implementation project is stressed by distributing over 40% of the SDLC on managing requirements.

The main activities of the Requirements Management are to meet the VOC and keep updated the Requirements Specification during the SDLC. The quality and completeness of the requirements contribute to the accuracy of the specification.

The success of computer systems implementation/maintenance depends on these three tasks. A practical and accurate Requirements Specification will contribute to the successful implementation of the computer system, on time, within the budget, and on schedule.

Requirements Management can achieve the success described above if it is maintained throughout the system lifecycle.

TOOLS

Tools noted here do not represent an endorsement but rather a sampling of tools in the category of requirements management. In most cases, tool names are trademarked by their respective developers.

Cybernetic Intelligence GmbH - EasyRM, http://www.cybernetic.org/contents/en/easyrm.php.

IBM Rational® RequisitePro® - IBM tool used for Requirements Management. https://www.ibm.com/support/knowledgecenter/en/SSSHCT_7.1.0/com.ibm.reqpro.help/helpindex_rp.html.

Rational Software – Rational RequisitePro, ftp://ftp.software.ibm.com/software/rational/web/datasheets/reqpro.pdf.

Siemens - Systems Engineering and Requirements https://www.plm.automation.siemens.com/en/products/teamcenter/requirements-management/

Telelogic Inc. - the tool used for Requirements Management http://www-01.ibm.com/software/awdtools/doors/?&ca=qapromo-s0swg-b0swg-l0-d0swgmer-n0363-o0doors-g0usen/.

CORE PRINCIPLE

User Requirements Specifications should describe the required functions of the computerized system and be based on documented risk assessment and GMP impact. User requirements should be traceable throughout the lifecycle (EU Annex 11-4.4).

REFERENCES

[1] López, O., "Requirements Management," *Journal of Validation Technology*, May 2013.

[2] A stakeholder is anyone who has a stake in the successful outcome of the project – system owner(s), business managers, regulated end-users, quality assurance, software engineers, support people, and so forth.

[3] ASTM E 2500 – 13 - Standard Guide for Specification, Design, and Verification of Pharmaceutical and Biopharmaceutical Manufacturing Systems and Equipment, November 2013.

[4] Roger S. Pressman, "*Software Engineering: A Practitioner's Approach*," 7th ed., McGraw-Hill, NY.

[5] https://deepsource.io/blog/exponential-cost-of-fixing-bugs/

[6] Product Requirements – include high-level features or capabilities that the business team has committed to delivering to a customer. Product Requirements do not specify how the features or the qualifications will be designed.

[7] Specification - A document that specifies, in a complete, precise, verifiable manner, the requirements, design, behavior, or other characteristics of a system or component, and often, the procedures for determining whether these provisions have been satisfied.

[8] *Establish – define, document, and implement*. (21 CFR 820.3(k))

[9] Carnegie Mellon University, Software Engineering Institute, *Capability Maturity Model Integration (CMMI) for Software*, Rev 3.0.

ADDITIONAL READINGS

Additional regulatory or guidance references associated with this topic can be found at *PIC/S Guidance on Good Practices for Computerized Systems in Regulated "GxP" Environments* (PI 011-3), US FDA 21 CFR 211.68; US FDA 21 CFR 820.30(g), 21 CFR 820.70(i) and 21 CFR 11.10(a).

Best Practices in Requirements Engineer http://www.stickyminds.com/sitewide.asp?Function=edetail&ObjectType=ART&ObjectId=13169&tth=DYN&tt=siteemail&iDyn=37

http://en.wikipedia.org/wiki/Requirements_traceability.

IEEE Std 1233 - *Guide for Developing System Requirements Specifications*, 1998.

ISO 9001 - *Quality management systems – Requirements*, 2015.

ISO/IEC 12207 - *Systems and software engineering* — Software lifecycle processes, 2017.

ISO/IEC 9126 - *Software engineering - Product quality*, 2001.

ISPE/GAMP, "*GAMP Traceability for GxP Regulated Application*," Pharmaceutical Engineering, Vol 26 No 1, January/February 2006.

NASA – Software Engineering Documents, https://www.nasa.gov/offices/oce/functions/software/index.html.

US Center for Disease Control (CDC), "*Unified Process Practices Guide – Requirements Management*," UP Version 06/30/07. http://www2.cdc.gov/cdcup/.

US Food and Drugs Administration (FDA), *General Principles of Software Validation; Final Guidance for Industry and FDA Staff*, June 2001.

Chapter 5

INTEGRATION BETWEEN COMPUTER SYSTEMS AND E-RECORDS LIFECYCLES

INTRODUCTION

Ensuring that both SLCs are integrated, helps facilitate the development and implementation of more robust computer systems by reducing risks to operation. The system owner ensures that the system and data integrity teams are part of the SDLC activities.

Such a team's integration fosters and e-records increased cooperation among personnel responsible for the design, implementation, assessment, operation maintenance, and final disposition of the system and e-records.

Organizations maximize the use of system functionality, and e-records controls relevant information generated during the SDLC process to satisfy requirements for similar information needed for other systems and e-records integrity controls purposes.

Reusing requirements for similar systems and associated e-records integrity controls promote consistency of information during the assessments, development, operation, and maintenance.

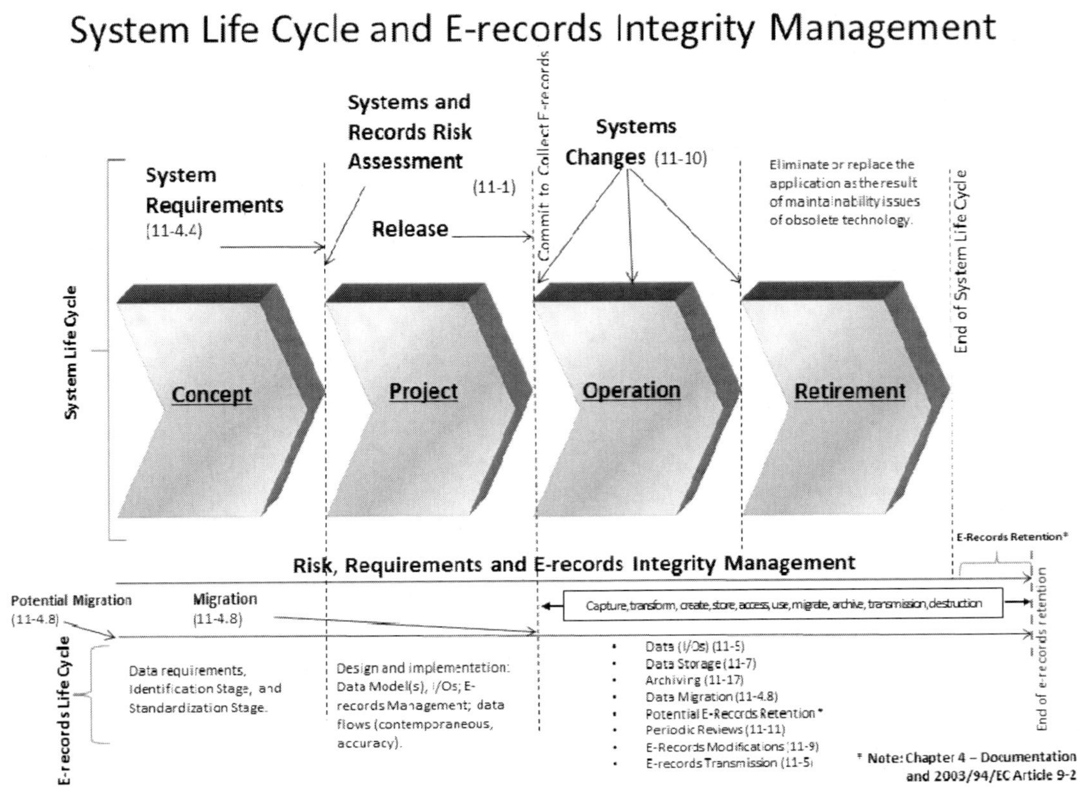

Figure 5.1. Integration between computer systems and E-records lifecycles.

After the computer system is released to operations, the prominence in the e-records is the management of the e-records during creation, transformation, access, using, migrating, storing, and disposal after the system is released. The typical CGMP controls associated with the Operational Period of the computer system take over. Comparable CGMP controls applicable to the computer systems apply to the e-records.

Figure 5.1 depicts an approach to integrating the e-records lifecycle during the system lifecycle (SLC). The selected SLC is from the EU Annex 11 [1].

E-records governance [2] is the computer systems validation (CSV) process. Besides, to demonstrate the quality embedded in the system during the SLC, this process provides the initial assurance of the successful implementation of the e-records integrity controls and the computer systems records management. These record controls are to be maintained through the operation and even after the retirement of the computer system.

CSV is the formal assessment and reporting of quality and performance measures for all the lifecycle stages of software and system development, its implementation, qualification and acceptance, operation, modification, re-qualification, maintenance, and retirement. This should enable both the regulated user and competent authority to have a high level of confidence in the integrity of both the processes executed within the controlling computer system(s) and in those processes controlled by and/or linked to the computer system(s), within the prescribed operating environment(s) [3].

In the context of worldwide health authority regulations, the validation process applicable to computer systems incorporates the intended purpose of the systems.

The SLC incorporates the CSV process.

Using the EU Annex 11, the following sections feature the integration between the computer systems and e-records lifecycles. The e-records lifecycle is discussed in Chapter 3.

CONCEPT PERIOD

The Concept Period establishes the definition of the project (EU Annex 11 p4.5 [1]), including precise data integrity goals and objectives, and the generation of the quality plan (EU Annex 11 p3 [1] and EU Annex 11 p4.5 [1]).

In addition to the above activities, during the Concept Period, the process is understood and system requirements (EU Annex 11 p4.4 [1]) delineated. The system requirements incorporate a system's configuration for a hardware and software application to run smoothly and efficiently. Failure to meet these requirements can result in installation, operational and/or performance challenges. The installation problems may prevent a device or application from getting installed. In contrast, performance problems may cause a product to malfunction, perform below expectation, or even hang or crash.

Non-functional requirements should be part of the system requirements as well.

From the context of the e-records lifecycle, it is incorporated two stages defining the planning, requirements and designing of the e-records model and the functionality to manage the e-records model. These are discussed in Chapter 3.

PROJECT PERIOD - RISK ASSESSMENT

A mature e-records governance system adopts a "quality risk management" approach across all areas of the quality system (EU Annex 11 p4.5 [1]).

During the Project Period, the process, system, and records risk assessments are performed. The objective of these assessments is to identify risks during the operation. These uncovered risks, if any, will be used to support the technological and procedural controls mitigating the risks.

The critical e-records are identified. The integrity risks to critical e-records will vary depending upon the degree to which the e-records generated by the computer system can be configured, and therefore potentially manipulated (EU Annex 11 p12.2 [1]). The other critical area to be considered is transient data during creating the e-records [2].

Other areas to be assessed are capture, transformation (as applicable), creation, storing, access, use, transmission, migration, archiving and final disposition to e-records.

An assessment of the risks of the e-records is performed to the areas described above, uncovering possible e-records manipulations in an unauthorized manner and, via a root analysis, finding the mitigation(s) to the potential unauthorized manipulation of the e-records. These analyses may lead to architecture and design tradeoffs during system design and development.

Refer to Chapter 14, E-records Vulnerabilities.

The MHRA guidance [6] suggests mitigations to address the risk of e-records manipulations in an unauthorized manner.

- Access controls to ensure that only authorized individuals can access and use the system based on the job role (EU Annex 11 p12 [1]). The access controls apply to database servers or any server containing GMP related e-records.
- The regulated entity must have documentation about users and access level (EU Annex 11 p12.3 [1]). This documentation must be consistent with the actual access settings in the system.
- In cases that technological or design constraints don't allow unique access to the computer application and/or database server(s), a procedural control must provide access and traceability.
- The access to system administrators should be minimal, unique per administrator and traceable. The preferred traceability method for actions performed by a system administrator is audit trails (EU Annex 11 p9 [1]). EU Annex 11 [1] does not specify if the audit trails must be electronically recorded.

- Separation of roles must be enforced on e-records maintenance.
- E-records maintenance must be controlled (EU Annex 11 p12.4 [1]) and an approval method must be implemented (EU Annex 11 p10 [1]).

Another area to consider is the risk of e-records migration from an existing system(s) over to a new system [4]. The risk of e-records migration may be mitigated by verifying "that data is not altered in value and/or meaning during this migration process" (EU Annex 11 p4.8 [1]).

As described in Chapter 6 in this book, Annex 20 [5] summarizes an approach to quality risk management pertinent to computer systems and computer-controlled equipment. The risks uncovered during this activity must be managed through the SLC (EU Annex 11 p1 [1]).

The e-records risk management must be performed during the e-records lifecycle (EU Annex 11 p1 [1]). Before starting the design, as part of the Project Stage, of the computer system and/or the e-records management function, decisions regarding well-known risks.

According to the MHRA guidance [6], "the effort and resource assigned to data governance should be commensurate with the risk to product quality."

Besides, the MHRA communicated to the regulated user that they must carry out a routine effectiveness review of their governance systems to ensure that e-records integrity and traceability are maintained [7]. The effectiveness review can be performed during the periodic review.

The requirements document must include a requirement(s) related to mitigating the uncovered risks.

Manufacturers must develop and use a system that allows an acceptable risk.

PROJECT PERIOD – REQUIREMENTS

Business requirements are gathered as part of the Concept Phase at the beginning of the computer system project, including the e-records integrity-related requirements. These e-records integrity-related requirements are traced to the regulated entity e-records governance (EU Annex 11 p4.4 [1]).

The following e-records integrity requirements are critical:

- Identify critical data and e-records.
- Develop a data flow diagram.
- Establish e-records management requirements (e.g., e-records written contemporaneously).
- Establish the criteria related to transient data (e.g., security).
- Identify interfaces (EU Annex 11 p5 [1]) and the data to be entered manually (EU Annex 11 p6 [1]).
- Develop data models and databases.
- The data flow diagram and risk assessment, identify the e-records integrity-related controls. The identified risk must be managed through the SLC (EU Annex 11 p1 [1]).
- Suppose e-records from a legacy system and/or any other system are migrated to the system under development. In that case, there must be a verification to demonstrate that the e-records value and/or meaning have not been altered. This verification must include associated metadata.
- Based on risk assessment, assess the need for audit trails (EU Annex 11 p12.4 [1]), and controls to prevent unauthorized access to the application, servers and the operating systems (EU Annex 11p 7.1 [1], EU Annex 11 p12 [1] and 21 CFR 11.10(g)).
- Identify and protect the reliable time source that is to be used to generate timestamps.
- Identify storage, archiving, and migration needs.

The appropriate methods to prevent unauthorized manipulation of e-records include:

- use of keys.
- passwords.
- personal codes.
- restricted access to computer terminals.

Of particular interest are the system administrator access and the access to the e-records retained by computer storage (EU Annex 11 p7.1 [1]). According to the MHRA guidance [6], MHRA expects each system administrator to have unique access to the computer system appropriate for their job role. Every regulated user with administrative privileges is logged into the computer system with distinct log attributes. This distinctiveness ensures traceability of actions performed in the computer and the respective user, including an audit trail. This exception may not apply to read-only activities.

During the development period of a new system in which a legacy system is replaced, the requirements stage must consider the e-records migration from the legacy system to the new system. If this is the case, it will require:

- considering storage and infrastructure requirements.
- mapping source and destination fields.
- specification of the mandatory fields for e-records.
- extracting and loading requirements.
- specifications of the e-records inputs (e.g., format, decimal places, units, ranges, limits, defaults, and the conversion requirements).
- defining what constitutes an error and how errors must be handled.
- verification requirements to ensure that source e-records are the same as the e-records in the destination.

As the reader can conclude the above requirements, this is a project by itself.

The business requirements are transformed into user requirements or capabilities needed to solve or achieve an objective. Finally, the user requirements are translated to functional requirements or requirements that specific computer system behaviour or functions (EU Annex 11 p4.4 [1]).

With the information collected until this instant in the project, a supplier may be contemplated to carry out the design.

Project Period – Building, Testing, Documenting and Installing

As part of the Project Period and based on the solution architecture, the application is built, tested, and tested and documented, installed, and deployed.

The requirements are translated into configurations and design controls to manage the identified risks, including e-records integrity risks.

The following is addressed by the EU Annex 11 [1] guideline:

- IT infrastructure must be qualified to ensure capacity, security and e-records integrity (EU Annex 11-Principle b [1]).
- As part of the qualification of the application and associated controls, test the backup and restoration procedure(s), and verify the output of the backup (EU Annex 11 p7.2 [1]). Each backup set should be checked to ensure error-free, including the metadata and all configuration related files.
- The ability to retrieve the e-records and audit trails should be ensured and tested (EU Annex 11 p7.1 [1]).
- Verify the accuracy of reports and audit trail reports (EU Annex 11 p8 [1]).

- As applicable, and based on the operational sequencing, test accuracy of the e-records (EU Annex 11 p7.1 [1]) and workflows.
- The level of access is assigned based on the duties of each user (EU Annex 11 p2 [1]).
- Training related to the operational aspect of the system is a relevant element of the proper operation of the system.

Data flows and mappings are reviewed during the design of the system.

PROJECT PERIOD - E-RECORDS MIGRATION AND COMPUTER SYSTEMS RELEASE TO OPERATIONS

Suppose e-records are transferred to a new environment changing the format of the e-records. In that case, the qualification must include test cases and the associated verifications that the electronic records new format do not alter the content of the records and associated metadata during the migration process (EU Annex 11 p4.8 [1]). The migrated records and the application(s) are integrated, and testing is executed to demonstrate integration [4].

As part of the implementation, one of many e-records integrity-related requirements addressed in the MHRA guideline [6] is recording transactions contemporaneously by computer systems. These are typical transactions where the user agrees, completes by performing specific pre-defined actions or acknowledges a deviation. These actions must not be combined into a single computer system transaction with other operations.

The above guideline can be traced to Section 4.8 in Volume 4, Chapter 4 (Documentation) from the EudraLex "Rules Governing Medicinal Products in the European Union".

"Records should be made or completed at the time each action is taken and in such a way that all significant activities concerning the manufacture of medicinal products are traceable."

Recording e-records contemporaneously is a key factor related to e-records reliability.

Operations Periods

During this stage, e-records are generated, transformed, recorded, accessed, used, integrated, logically deleted, migrated, and retired. It is when the integrity of the e-records can be compromised. The objective of all e-records requirements, and the implementation of such requirements, are to preserve the e-records integrity.

During the operational stage the procedural controls associated with e-records integrity must be enforced:

- only authorized people can modify the e-records stored on data servers or any other media.
- there is a record of changes made.
- the entry of e-records considered critical are checked by a designated person other than the one who made the records or checked by the system itself.
- availability of a procedural control for cancellation changes to the level of approval and for entering or editing e-records, including changing of personal passwords.

The e-records integrity controls can be categorized in four spaces: e-records created, e-records in storage, e-records during processing, and e-records while in transit [8]. These controls impact the computer system during the operational phase.

Computer System Retirement – E-Records Migration

The activities to migrate e-records as part of a computer system retirement are not different from the migration of e-records as part of the transfer of e-records to a new computer system, discussed previously.

E-records must be preserved as part of the planning to retire the computer system generating e-records.

The e-records preservation plan must include one of the following options:

- Make sure that a new system will be able to retrieve e-records from previous systems.
- Preserve previous applications (not contemplated, the system is to be retired).
- Archive hard copies (when allowed).
- Completion of system documentation and validation dossier.

If archiving hard copies, computer records reproduced in paper copies is the selected method to migrate the e-records, the paper copies must be certified as true copies of the original e-records, and the paper copies are to be signed and dated as verified true copies. All electronic metadata must be part also part of the fixed record. The verified hard copy must then be stored with other paper-based records.

After executing the e-records preservation plan, ensure that the regulated user's quality assurance (QA) unit performs an audit on the preserved records. The audit will verify the traceability between planning and implementation and assess the preservation plan's successful execution.

E-records migration must protect e-records from deliberate or accidental alteration or loss [9].

E-RECORDS ARCHIVING

In the context of e-records no longer actively required, these e-records can be archived. This is considered an extended retention environment.

E-records archiving is the process of moving e-records that are no longer actively used to a separate records storage device for long-term retention, often disabling the e-records from any further changes. The retention period of these e-records has not been finalized.

The controls applicable to e-records in storage are also applicable to archived records.

The archiving process is an activity that may involve a modification of format, media, and/or physical storage. It must be performed in a controlled manner following a procedural control.

There are multiple types of archiving disposition:

- Extract/Migrate – The migration of digital information from one hardware/software configuration to another or from one generation of computer technology to a later one offers one method of dealing with technological obsolescence. Data is extracted from the current system and moved to another location, or the entire instance is migrated elsewhere.
- Host – These are single-instance database systems that are not typically managed by the site and are hosted elsewhere.
- Archive – Will contain the following types:
  - Report – the official record is in hard copy, or the most effective end state will become hard copy.
  - Physical to virtual (P2V) (Encapsulate) – To be able to access the e-record effectively, in some cases, it is necessary to have both the application and the database in a virtual environment. Encapsulation is a technique for grouping together a digital object and anything else necessary to provide access to that object. In this case, the software will

be used to encapsulate the data and application and the product housed in a server designated for this purpose.

- Technology emulation creates an environment that behaves in a hardware-like manner. It potentially offers substantial benefits in preserving the functionality and integrity of digital objects.
- Keeping every version of software and hardware – the requirement for keeping every version of software and hardware, operating systems and manuals, and the retention of personnel with the relevant technical skills. This option makes preserving obsolete technologies to access the archived e-records unfeasible.

Suppose the e-records in storage are transferred to another format, media or system. In that case, the archiving process must include verifications that the e-records are not altered in value and/or meaning during this migration process. The metadata must also be transferred and verified. Refer to "Data Migration" in this chapter.

The computer system holding the archived records must implement all security-related functions to restrict access to authorized personnel only. Periodically, archived records need to be verified for accessibility, readability, integrity, and the state of security control.

If changes are implemented to the computer infrastructure and/or application, it is required to ensure and test the application's ability to access the e-records.

E-records may be retained on archived media for a very long period. The procedure addressing the e-records in storage should also address the stability of the storage media itself.

The records can be physically deleted after completing the specified record retention requirements.

Each country has its particularity about each best practice discussed in this book. One example of such particularity is the clinical e-records archiving guidelines established in South Africa. In South Africa, e-records must be reproduced in hard copy, which is to be signed and dated as a verified accurate copy of the original data. The verified hard copy should then be stored with other paper-based records. This requirement in South Africa is established to overcome the possibility of loss or inability to read the information due to technological redundancy.

The MHRA guidance [6] recommends that archive e-records be locked to not be altered or deleted without detection and audit trail.

The archive arrangements must be designed to permit recovery and readability of the e-records and metadata throughout the required retention period.

E-Records Final Disposition

The explanation of the e-records final disposition is contained in Chapter 3. Chapter 10 describes the requirements associated with the e-records final disposition.

References

[1] Computerized systems. In: The rules governing medicinal products in the European Union. Volume 4: Good manufacturing practice (GMP) guidelines: Annex 11. Brussels: European Commission. (http://ec.europa.eu/enterprise/pharmaceuticals/eudralex/vol-4/pdfs-en/anx11en.pdf).

[2] López, O., "*Defining and Managing Raw Manufacturing Data*," Pharmaceutical Technology, Vol 43 No 6, July 2019.

[3] PI 011-3. "*Good Practices for Computerized Systems in Regulated "GXP" Environments*," Pharmaceutical Inspection Cooperation Scheme (PIC/S), September 2007.

[4] López, O., "*E-records Migration and its Integrity*," Ensuring the Integrity of Electronic Health Records, (Routledge, Boca Raton, FL, 1st ed., 2021), pp. 121-124.

[5] *EudraLex, The Rules Governing Medicinal Products in the European Union*, Volume 4, EU Guidelines to Good Manufacturing Practice Medicinal Products for Human and Veterinary Use, Annex 20 - Quality Risk Management, February 2008.

[6] MHRA, *'GXP' Data Integrity Guidance and Definitions*, March 2018.

[7] MHRA, "*MHRA expectation regarding self-inspection and data integrity*," September 2014.

[8] López, O., "*Data Integrity in Pharmaceutical and Medical Devices Regulation Operations: Best Practices Guide to Electronic Records Compliance,*" CRC Press, Boca Ratón, Fl., 2017.

[9] López, O., "*E-records Migration and Its Integrity*," Ensuring the Integrity of Electronic Health Records, (Routledge, Boca Ratón, FL, 1st ed., 2021), pp. 121-124.

Chapter 6

CGMP E-RECORDS RISK MANAGEMENT [1]

INTRODUCTION

Risk Management is the systematic application of quality management policies, procedures, and practices to assess, control, communicate and review risk [2].

In the context of this book, e-records integrity is the property that the e-records have not been altered in an unauthorized manner [2]. E-records integrity service maintains e-records precisely as inputted and is auditable to affirm its reliability. As a function related to security, e-records integrity service protects from unauthorized modification (accidental or intentional), destruction, or disclosure [4].

The e-records risk management looks for possible e-records vulnerabilities (Chapter 14), mitigations, and the associated solutions to drive e-records from being lost, obscured or modified without a trace and ensures that activities are recorded at the time of performance (see 21 CFRs 211.68, 211.100, 211.160(a), 211.188, and 211.194).

The basis for the e-records risk management is the CGMP e-records requirement, including the good documentation practices.

NIST SP 800-39 [5] identifies four distinct steps for risk management. Risk management requires organizations to frame, assess, respond to, and monitor risks.

- Framing risk – describes how the regulated entities establish a risk context for e-records integrity. The purpose of the risk framing component is to produce a risk management strategy that addresses how the regulated entities intend to assess, respond to, and monitor Risk - while making clear and transparent the risk perceptions that regulated entities routinely use in making operational decisions. The framing is established typically as part of the governance document. This document ensures controls are in place to prevent and detect data integrity issues throughout the SLC and e-records lifecycle [5].
- Assessing risk – describes how the regulated entity analyzes risk within the context of the regulated entity risk frame. The purpose of the data integrity risk assessment component is to identify vital high-level risks to patient safety, product quality and data integrity and identify the required controls to manage those risks. Typically, at this stage, no assumptions are made about the nature or exact functionality and design of the computerized system(s) that will support the process.
- Responding to risk – addresses how the regulated user responds to risk once that risk is determined based on risk assessments. The purpose of the risk response component is to provide a consistent, organization-wide response to risk following the organizational risk frame by (i) developing alternative courses of action for responding to risk; (ii) evaluating the alternative courses of action; (iii) determining appropriate courses of action consistent with organizational risk tolerance; and (iv) implementing risk responses based on selected courses of action.

- Monitor Risk - Risk monitoring provides organizations with the means to (i) verify compliance, (ii) determine the ongoing effectiveness of risk response measures, and (iii) identify risk-impacting changes to organizational information systems and environments of operation. Analyzing monitoring results gives organizations the capability to maintain awareness of the risk being incurred, highlight the need to revisit other steps in the risk management process, and initiate process improvement activities as needed

The general principles of good documentation practices apply to the handling of records regardless of media (e.g., paper records or electronic records), throughout its lifecycle from the time data is first generated and any modifications made after that [6].

Quality Risk Management for Computer Systems

International Conference for Harmonization (ICH) Q9 [2] summarizes an approach to Quality Risk Management pertinent to determine the extent of validation to the computer systems and computer-controlled equipment.

- identification of critical performance parameters
- selection of the requirements and design
- code review
- the extent of testing and test methods
- reliability of electronic records and signatures

Risk Management [7, 8]

Risk management is integral to the e-records handling process. It is the driven process of digital transformation.

Risk management is about identifying the risks to the compliance area and understanding the impact of the risk.

Annex 20 [9] summarizes an approach to Quality Risk Management pertinent to computer systems and computer-controlled equipment.

- Determine the CGMP criticality of the system, impact on patient safety, product quality or e-records integrity; identification of the critical performance parameters; determine the extent of validation.
- Develop requirement specification considering the basis of the criticality; perform a detailed risk assessment to determine critical functions.
- Select of the design of computer hardware and software (e.g., modular, structured, fault tolerance); implementation of appropriate controls via design as much as possible.
- Perform code review and data flows, as applicable.
- Determine the extent of testing and test methods of the controls implemented during the design.
- Evaluate the reliability of e-records and signatures, as applicable.
- The risks uncovered during this activity must be managed through the SLC (EU Annex 11 p1).

The risk management process supports the assessment against the computer requirements and within its operational environment. Decisions regarding risks identified must be made before starting the design of the computer system.

According to the MHRA guidance [10], "the effort and resource assigned to data governance should be commensurate with the risk to product quality."

Below it can be found an example of the controls based on the impact to the e-records on patient safety, product safety and compliance.

Control	No Impact	Indirect Impact	Direct Impact
Access Control	• controlled access	• authorization process • access management • password management • documentation	• rigorous authorization control • strict and proactive access management • user profiles • unique accounts • stringent PW management • physical security • - full documentation
Backup and restore	• checking of outcome • Multiple copies (redundancy)	• Checking of outcome • Multiple copies (redundancy) • Formal periodic testing • Documentation	• Checking of outcome • Multiple copies (redundancy) • Formal periodic testing • Full documentation • Remote storage locations • - Automated processes

Risk mitigation strategies, like the above, need the understanding of many factors, including [11]:

- The degree to which e-records can be configured
- Understanding system complexity
- User access permissions, system configuration
- Transaction windows
- Understanding e-records structure
  - Dynamic vs static e-records
  - Access, security and hosting of e-records
  - File structure
- Validation for intended purpose vs functional verification
- Audit trails and metadata

The selected mitigation strategy (ies) will determine the associated controls. Integrating the SLC and risk management is essential to effectively implement and maintain the e-records integrity controls.

As part of the assessment of the risks associated with the possible issues about e-records integrity, failure analysis is performed to determine where the loss of e-records integrity would have the greatest impact, including the regulated entity reputation.

One of the tools to be used to perform the failure analysis is the data flow diagram. The data flow is a diagram that maps the flow of information of any process or system. The data or e-record can be in one of the following states: creation, in storage, during processing or while in transit.

Centered on the failure analysis results, the combination of techniques to be used, and the effort to implement and maintain an e-records integrity control(s) is based on the above states.

It is essential to review the risks periodically and if appropriate mitigation systems are revised. The effectiveness of a risk management process depends on the quality of information fed into the risk assessment process, which in turn relies on the robustness of the quality system in place.

Failure to manage e-records integrity risks can have the following impact:

- Authorization, completeness, and accuracy of transactions may be incorrect as they are entered, processed, summarized, and reported.
- There may be inadequate handling controls concerning the integrity of processed e-records or databases, which ultimately may affect the quality of a product.

Should be communicated the e-records integrity risks throughout the e-records lifecycle.

Regulatory Agencies Expectations

Two primary principles of quality risk management are [1] expected by the regulatory agencies:

- The quality risk evaluation should be based on scientific knowledge and ultimately link to the protection of the patient.
- The level of effort, formality and documentation of the quality risk management process should be commensurate with the level of risk.

REFERENCES

[1] López, O., "*CGMP E-Records Risk Assessments*," Journal of GXP Compliance, Vol. 22, Issue 5, September 2018.

[2] ICH Harmonized Tripartite Guideline, "*Quality Risk Management*, Q9", November 2005.

[3] NIST, "*Systems Security Engineering: Considerations for a Multidisciplinary Approach in the Engineering of Trustworthy Secure Systems*," (Special Publication 800-160 Vol 1), June 2004.

[4] Committee on National Security Systems Instruction (CNSSI), "*Glossary*," CNSSI 4009, April 2015.

[5] NIST, "*Managing Information Security Risk*," (Special Publication 800-39), March 2011.

[6] Health Canada, "*Good manufacturing practices guide for drug products*, GUI-0001," February 2018 (Version 3).

[7] NIST, "*An Introduction to Computer Security: The NIST Handbook*", Chapter 6, Computer Security Risk Management (Special Publication 800-12 Rev. 1), June 2017.

[8] Graham, L., "*Compliance matters, Good laboratory practice*," Blog MHRA Inspectorate, September 2015.

[9] *EudraLex, The Rule Governing Medicinal Products in the European Union*, Volume 4, EU Guidelines for Good Manufacturing Practices for Medicinal Products for Human and Veterinary Use, Annex 20, Quality Risk Management, February 2008.

[10] MHRA, "*GxP Data Integrity Guidance and Definitions*," March 2018.

[11] Churchward, D., "*GMP Compliance and Data Integrity*," paper presented at the PDA/PIC's Quality and Regulations Conference, Brussels, Belgium, June 2015.

ADDITIONAL READING

CEFIC, "*Practical Risk-based Guide for Managing Data Integrity*," March 2019 (Rev 1).

Chapter 7

SUPPORTING SERVICES

INTRODUCTION

Except Requirement #6, the requirements in this chapter are related to the design and implementation of e-records integrity governance.

The e-records governance refers to an organizational structure that includes written policies and procedures documenting processes to prevent and detect situations that may have an impact on e-records integrity.

Regulated companies should implement organizational structures to ensure that responsible systems and data are appropriately allocated, and duties are undertaken. The e-records governance should address data ownership throughout the data lifecycle.

The reader can notice the relevance of this chapter of the system owner and e-records owner [1]. From the context of e-records, the system owner is responsible for the security of the e-records residing on the repository for e-records (EU Annex 11, Glossary [2]).

Requirement #6 provides technical guidance to vendors in creating e-records management tools and specifications for regulated entities to consider when procuring them.

E-Records Lifecycle Requirements

The following e-records supporting services requirements maintain the e-records integrity as part of the e-records lifecycle.

Requirement 1 - *The e-records owner [1] must manage all e-records, including all recorded information, regardless of form or characteristics, made or received by the regulated entity as evidence of a regulated activity of the regulated entity.*

E-records must be generated and maintained under the oversight of a pharmaceutical quality system that ensures their accuracy [3].

Organizations must establish a data governance system to address data ownership and ensure controls are in place to prevent and detect data integrity issues throughout the e-records lifecycle [2]. Refer to Chapter 3.

The data governance program must refer to policies and procedures addressing data management. Furthermore, the elements of effective management governance should include: the data governance considers the design, operation, and monitoring of processes/systems to comply with the principles of data integrity, including control over intentional and unintentional changes to data [4].

The e-records under the medicines' manufacturing practices regulations are properly managed regardless of storage media or other characteristics.

Requirement 2 - *The e-records owner must regularly monitor and review access rights and permission rules for e-records; these rules should be updated as applicable.*

As a function related to security e-records, integrity service maintains the e-records in an original format as the original record. Records should be traceable to the source the record was generated to affirm its reliability.

One of the main controls to maintain the reliability of the e-records must include that all access and user rights in electronic systems are properly controlled to prevent system users from compromising data integrity. The review of user access rights shall be performed periodically based on the criticality of the e-records. The periodic review verifies the effectiveness of the implemented procedural and technological control measures.

As part of the periodic review or self-inspection [4], the security of the data servers and associated operating system is evaluated to confirm that the security controls remain in a valid state and are compliant with CGMP. These controls must prevent manipulation and/or unscheduled destruction of raw e-records.

It is verified the effectiveness of existing control measures to the data server and considered the possibility of unauthorized activity at all interfaces.

The periodic review considers assessing users' access to users changing jobs.

The System Administrator rights should not be assigned to users with a direct interest in the data.

Requirement 3 - *E-records owner users should regularly monitor and evaluate their records controls.*

The e-records owner must periodically monitor data integrity issues with a corrective and preventive action plan (CAPA) to address identified issues [5]. It includes regularly assessing the effectiveness of the implemented preventative measures.

Periodically, a system review shall evaluate the current range of functionality, deviation records, incidents, changes, problems, upgrade history, performance, reliability, manual check of the system access log, security, automated notification of lockouts, and validation status reports. The period shall be defined based on risk.

The incidents and their resolutions shall be tracked to monitor the performance of both the process and the electronic system within which the incident occurred. This traceability usually is done using an incident log [6].

As part of the periodic reviews, there shall be regular management reviews of quality metrics related to data integrity.

Quality metrics shall address the following type of actions [6]:

- Preventive, oriented to oversee the rules expected to prevent Integrity failures (e.g., Operators/Supervisor Data Integrity Awareness Rate, Sample Turn Around Time)
- Corrective, oriented to monitor the completion and outcome of records compliance vs ALCOA+ requirements (e.g., Electronic Records Assessed Rate, Integrity Corrective Action Rate)
- Monitoring, oriented to supervise the number of actual integrity failures and the relevant follow up (e.g., Data Integrity Internal Verification Rate, Spontaneous Integrity Failures Rate, i.e., Reported by operators)

These metrics are intended to demonstrate management commitment to ensure the integrity of CGMP data management.

Requirement 4 - *The e-records owner retains the responsibility for managing their e-records, regardless of whether they reside in a service provider.*

Data integrity relating to a product or process may cross various boundaries within the lifecycle. From the organizational context:

- Internal (e.g., between production, QC and QA)
- External (e.g., between contract givers and acceptors)
- Cloud-based applications and storage

Cloud and External computing services are to be treated as a contracted service, with risks identified and addressed, responsibilities clearly outlined in a contract or service agreement and, ownership, retrieval, retention and security of data.

Internal IT departments of a regulated company should be considered external (EU Annex 11-3.1 [2]). In this case, a service agreement must be established.

The responsibilities of the contract giver and acceptor should be defined in a technical agreement or contract. Upon request, it should ensure timely access to data (including metadata and audit trails) to the data owner and competent national authorities. Contracts with providers should define archiving and continued readability of the data throughout the retention period (see archive).

Appropriate arrangements must exist to restore the software/system as per its original validated state, including validation and change control information to permit this restoration.

Business continuity arrangements should be included in the contract and tested. The need for an audit of the service provider should be based on risk [3].

The reliability of the electronic systems operated by the regulated user is always under the responsibility of the system owner, which shall document the relevant validation process leveraging the documentation provided by the cloud service provider or, internally, by the validation team.

The system owner is always the owner of the CGMP e-records.

Requirement 5 - *The system owner or representative must have controls to prevent unauthorized use, alteration, suppression, or deletion of records. Examples of controls include audit trails, access lists, monitoring, and periodic reviews.*

Ensure that all access and user rights to the electronic systems are properly controlled to prevent unauthorized users from compromising data integrity [2].

Additional technical controls are required to avoid authorized and unauthorized users compromising data integrity when the data is in storage.

An essential technical control to e-records changes is the audit trails. The objective of audit trails is to keep a record of the changes to the e-records performed by the users. The audit trail will provide forward and backward traceability. To track the audit trails, a reliable timestamp to each modification of a record is included. The audit trail should include changes made to the record, who made the change, the time and date the record was changed, and, if applicable, the reason the record was modified [3].

For critical data entered manually, there should be an additional check on the accuracy of the data. This check may be done by a second operator or by a validated electronic system (EU Annex 11 p6 [2]).

Electronic systems exchanging data electronically with other systems should include appropriate built-in checks for the correct and secure entry and processing of data to minimize data integrity risks (EU Annex 11 p5 [2]).

Built-in checks verification methods may include the use of [7]:

- Secure transfer
- Encryption
- Checksums

Where applicable, interfaces between systems should be designed and qualified to include an automated data transfer.

The EU Annex 11 p5 [2] built-in checks guideline is equivalent to the US FDA compliance policy guide (CPG) 7132a.07, Input/Output (I/O) checking guideline. I/O checks of data, as required by US FDA 21 CFR 211.68, are necessary to assure the data accuracy passing by the interfaces of two or more computers.

The other sources of possible e-records loss are the move of active e-records and archiving e-records.

Transferring active e-records from the current processing environment to another environment or migration can be performed by verifying the e-records in the migrated repository are not altered from the source repository in value and/or meaning. The migrated records must contain the data and associated metadata in the source repository. These migrated e-records should be original or compatible with the original structure.

Moving e-records from the processing environment to the retention environment or archiving is performed to safekeeping and preservation of the e-records after the e-records are inactive, superseded, replaced, or withdrawn from use. Typically, these e-records are preserved with view only attribute.

Backups at regular intervals are another relevant control to protect against potential data loss due to system issues or data corruption. US FDA 21 CFR Part 211.68 requires that the "backup data are exact and complete." The terms exact and complete refers that the backup data must be precise, complete, and secure from alteration, unintended erasures, or loss. The backup file should contain the data (including associated metadata) and should be in the original format or compatible with the original format [8].

Requirement 6 - *Regulated users must be responsible for monitoring changes to third-party terms of service that may affect records management.*

The management of e-records is the process of ensuring that e-records are stored, archived, or disposed of safely and securely during the e-records lifecycle.

Where the system owner chooses to outsource the storage of e-records (e.g., DaaS, SaaS), which can affect product conformity with requirements, the system owner shall ensure control and hold responsibility for the suitability and operability over such computer-related service. Control of such outsourced computer-related services shall be identified within the quality management system [9] and a clear statement of the responsibilities of the cloud service provider. The duties information is defined in a formal quality agreement (e.g., Service Level Agreement (SLA)).

Any service provided by a third party must be monitored and evaluated (ISO 15489-1:2016(E)). Any changes to the management of e-records without the revision and approval in the SLA may create reliability issues to the e-records.

Changes in terms of services must be discussed with the regulated user before implementation. Any agreement between the regulated user and the service provider must be implemented and approved in the SLA.

REFERENCES

[1] *Data Ownership - The allocation of responsibilities for data control to a specific process owne*r. (PIC/S))

[2] EudraLex, The Rules Governing Medicinal Products in the European Union, Volume 4, "EU Guidelines to Good Manufacturing Practice, Medicinal Products for Human and Veterinary Use Part 1, Annex 11 - Computerized Systems," June 2011

[3] Health Canada, "*Good manufacturing practices guide for drug products, GUI-0001,*" February 2018 (Version 3).

[4] MHRA, "*GxP Data Integrity Guidance and Definitions,*" March 2018.

[5] CEFIC, "*Practical risk-based guide for managing data integrity,*" March 2019 (Version 1).

[6] Federal State Institute of Drugs and Good Practices (FSI SID & GP, "*Data Integrity & Computer System Validation,*" August 2018.

[7] PIC/S PI 041-1, "*Good Practice for Data Management and Integrity in Regulated GMP GDP Environments,*" July 2021.

[8] US FDA, "*Data Integrity and Compliance with Drug CGMP - Questions and Answers, Guidance for Industry*," December 2018.

[9] ISO 9001, *Quality Management Systems – Requirements* (Section 4.1).

Chapter 8

Generation, Capture or Recording of Raw Data

Introduction

The typical way to create an e-record is by writing on media to render the data in a human-readable form.

Data is created, for example, in process automation after the instrument/equipment interfacing with an electronic system by issuing electrical signals in analogue form. These analogue signals must convert the analogue to digital signals for use by the electronic system. To convert to digital signals, signal converter devices are used. In Figure 8.1, these transformations are represented by the I/O card. The digital signal is converted to a data point after it is saved to a repository for e-records under records management control for disposition and access purposes.

As an example, in a Big Data environment, data can be created by combining two or more data points. This transformation refers to the cleansing and aggregation that may need to happen to data to prepare it for analysis. The combined data points are considered a data point after it is saved to a repository for e-records under records management control for disposition and access purposes.

Data is collected when e-records are imported from other sources, manually entered into the system, or linked to other systems. After being collected, the data point is placed under records management control for disposition and access purposes. The data points are not necessarily moved from the system they reside in when they are captured.

Besides, the collected data needs to be recorded immediately after generating, collecting, and/or transforming (21 CFR 211.100). These records collected after the data is generated, collected, and/or transformed are also original (21 CFR 211.180).

When the record contains CGMP data, the record becomes a CGMP record.

If the CGMP e-records are the first-capture e-records, the e-records are considered then CGMP raw e-records. Figure 8.1 collects data at the Supervisory Control and Data Acquisition (SCADA) or Historian level.

Some controls to collect data include [1]:

- The interface between the originating system, data acquisition and recording systems should be qualified to ensure the accuracy of data (21 CRF 211.68(b) or EU Annex 11 p5 [2]).
- Collected data can be saved into memory in a format that is not vulnerable to manipulation, loss, or change.
- The system software should incorporate checks to ensure the completeness of data acquired and any relevant metadata associated with the data (EU Annex 11 p5 [2]).

A record consists of generated, collected, and/or transformed individual data points treated as a unit. The generated, collected, and/or transformed e-records must ensure traceability, legibility and integrity of the generated, collected, and/or transformed data points. The generated, collected, and/or transformed data points must be defined and specified during the Data Process Design and addressed during the design process.

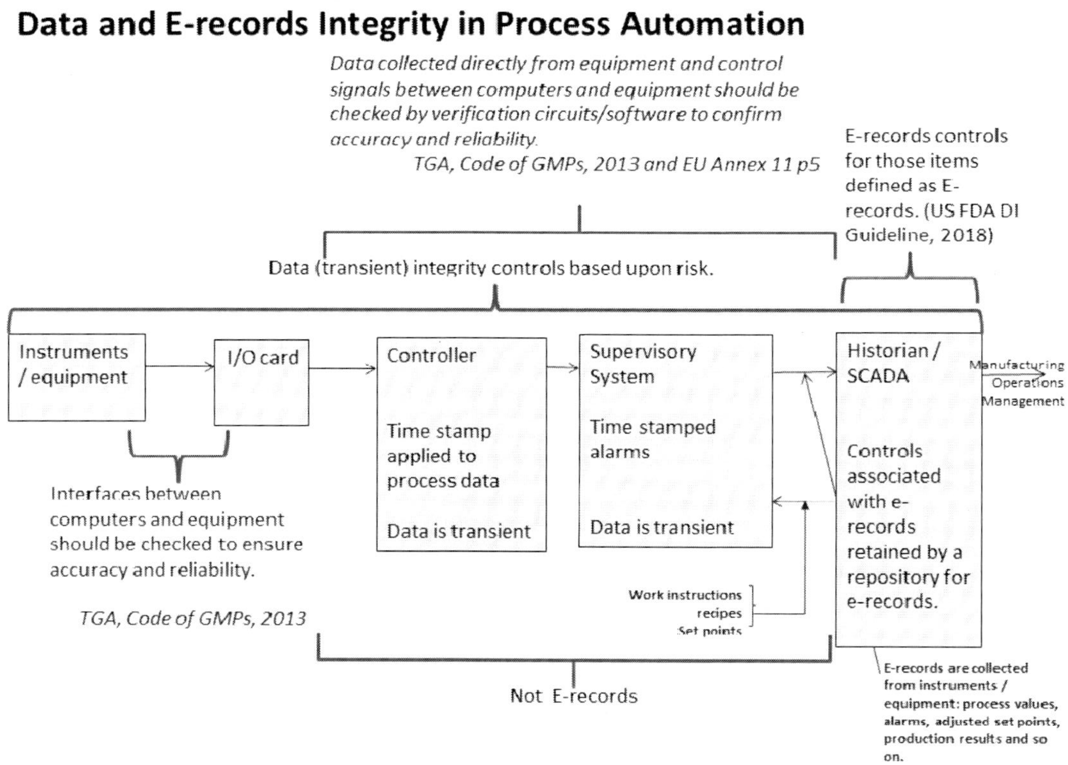

Figure 8.1. Data and E-records Integrity in Process Automation.

These data points must be defined and specified. Refer to Chapter 3, Records Identification Phase.

- The validation of the data handling process must cover the generation, collection, and transformation of data points. Each is the outcome of a qualified practice (qualified equipment, validated process or validated method). If data is transferred via interfaces, the authenticity and integrity of received data must be ensured. Manual interaction during data creation requires additional controls, including an additional check on the accuracy of the data (21 CRF 211.68(b) or EU Annex 11 p5 [2]).

This additional check can be done by a second operator or by a validated electronic means. Manual recording of critical values from display requires a secondary verification of the values entered before the e-records are committed.

This chapter provides and discusses data controls applicable to data generated, collected, and/or transformed.

The following aspects should be considered when determining risk and control measures [3]:

- Is it possible to recreate, amend or delete original data and metadata?
- How data is transferred to other locations or systems for processing or storage?

Data Capture and Creation Requirements

The following Data Capture and Creation requirements provide meaning for placing an object under records management control for disposition and access purposes.

***Requirement** 7 - An e-record must provide adequate and proper documentation of the CGMP requirement when generated to satisfy such requirement for as long as the information is needed.*

As part of the Data Processing Design in the e-records lifecycle, the CGMP information requirements are established. It is then analysed which is the most suitable method for getting the CGMP record(s) linked with the production process. This is performed by analyzing the input, processes, and output requirements. E-records planning identifies the CGMP e-records required to satisfy specific product/process quality requirements most efficiently.

The final product of the Data Processing Design is the approved standard e-records and metadata, including e-records entities, attributes, definitions, and values.

After the e-record is created, technological and procedural controls must be implemented to establish e-records integrity services to maintain information precisely as created. If the created e-record is modified an audit trail captures the modification allowing forward and backwards traceability.

Another control helping the reliability of e-records are the backups, security, and practical training to the regulated user.

The technological and procedural controls are required until the final disposition of the e-records.

***Requirement 8** - An e-record is considered reliable if it ensures a full and accurate representation of the transactions or activities.*

An e-record is reliable and accurate when the record symbolizes a full and precise representation of the transactions, activities or facts to which they attest and can be depended upon in the course of subsequent transactions or activities.

Data accuracy refers to whether the data values stored for an object are the correct values. To be corrected, data values must be the right value and must be represented in a consistent and unambiguous form.

The data accuracy is designed to minimize the risks to enter erroneous data. EU Annex 11 p5 [2] covers computers, instruments, or equipment interfaces. EU Annex 11 p6 [2] covers when the data is entered manually. In both cases, the objective of the built-in and accuracy checks, correspondingly, is the verification of the correctness of the collected data. During the EU Annex 11 [2] Project Phase, these accuracy-related workflows are tested and periodically verified during the EU Annex 11 [2] Operational Phase as part of the inputs and outputs (I/Os) verifications activities (21 CFR Part 211.68(b)).

Requirement 9 - *A record is considered reliable if it can be depended upon during subsequent transactions or activities.*

A reliable record is one whose contents can be trusted as a full and accurate representation of the transactions, activities, or facts to which they attest and can be depended upon in the course of subsequent transactions or activities.

These reliable records can be loaded to another e-records repository to be integrated, as an example, with another e-record.

If the e-records of the source systems are not reliable, such integration will not be reliable too.

The following aspects should be considered when assessing the reliability of e-records for subsequent transactions or activities [4]:

- How is data processed?
- How is data processing recorded?
- Is the data recorded contemporaneously?
- Does the person that processes the data influence what data is reported or how it is presented?

An element of a reliable e-record is its integrity. All e-records must be managed through the e-record lifecycle by an e-records handling service. This service must store, archive, and dispose of safely and securely e-records through its lifecycle.

As part of the e-records handling service, the e-records integrity service maintains the information exactly as it was created and is auditable to support the reliability.

Requirement 10 - *A record is considered to have integrity if it is complete and protected from unauthorized addition, deletion, alteration, use, and concealment.*

Completeness is the property of all necessary parts of the e-record in question. Complete data should be represented in the original context and associated metadata. Data profiling is required to assess the completeness of an e-record and establish the e-record structure and content. Loading data into the records structure as part of the creation of the e-records assess how the structure contains the allowed values. After consistently meeting the criteria of valid allowed values contained in the defined structure, the e-record can be designated as complete.

As a function related to security, e-records integrity service maintains information exactly as captured and created. If the e-records are modified/deleted after capture, an audit trail is generated to record the modification(s). To affirm the e-records reliability, any changes are auditable with bi-directional traceability.

Requirement 11 - *Security controls must be established for all computer systems as a means of ensuring e-records protection. Computer security is the principal enabler to create the integrity of e-records [5].*

To ensure integrity to the e-records, it is essential to assure trustworthy electronic systems. Trustworthy electronic systems are the first line of defence to protect the critical e-records managed by these systems.

Trustworthy electronic systems consist of computer infrastructure, applications, and procedures that:

- are reasonably suited to performing their intended functions
- provide a sufficiently reliable level of availability, reliability and correct operation
- are reasonably secure from intrusion and misuse
- adhere to generally accepted security principles

The driver of the electronic systems validation process is to ensure an acceptable degree of evidence (documented, raw data), confidence (dependability and thorough, rigorous achievement of predetermined specifications), intended use, accuracy, consistency and reliability [6], or that the electronic system is trustworthy.

In the context of e-records integrity, the objectives of a trustworthy electronic system are to ensure:

- consistency of data; in particular, preventing unauthorized creation, alteration, or destruction of data (Integrity)
- that legitimate users are not improperly denied access to information and resources (Availability)
- those resources are used only by authorized persons in authorized ways (Legitimate use)

Trustworthy electronic systems must be set up to ensure e-records protection against modification/deletions in an unauthorized manner.

Requirement 12 - *A record is considered usable if it can be located, retrieved, presented, and interpreted.*

E-records must be available during the period of retention. E-records must not only exist; they must be accessible. If the e-records are available, the e-records may be usable.

Usability is "the extent to which specified users can use a product to achieve specified goals with effectiveness, efficiency and satisfaction in a specified context of use" [7].

The definition by ISO establishes a structure for setting usability scope. The scope is operationally defined by specifying and target values for effectiveness, efficiency, and satisfaction. Measurements of these attributes enable comparing application progress over time and the comparison of multiple applications.

Effectiveness looks at the number of participants who can complete a task in a reasonable amount of time.

Efficiency is measured by the length of time required to complete a task.

Satisfaction consists of subjective measures regarding a user's perception of usability and evaluation.

Requirement 13 - *An authentic record is considered authoritative evidence of a transaction or event; records are accurate if they are what they claim to be.*

Care must be taken to ensure the authenticity of e-records.

An authentic e-record is what it intends to be. The authentic record is accordingly issued by an authorized person, regulated company, or authorized source. The requirements under Part 11.10 [8], are controls intended to ensure the authenticity and integrity of e-records.

Examples of these controls in Part 11.10 [8] are access controls, operational checks, validation to the systems managing the e-records, qualification of the infrastructure transporting the data, device checks, generation of accurate records; audit trails; records time stamping by system clock; training of users and electronic system developers, and so on.

As an example, the devise check is used to determine the validity of the source of data input (Part 11.10(h) [8]). It is warranted where only specific devices have been selected as legitimate data input sources. In such cases, the device checks would be used to determine if the data was authorized.

Another technological control protecting e-records authentication is encryption. Encryption does not itself prevent interference but denies the intelligible content to a would-be interceptor by encoding the information [9].

Requirement 14 - *A record must be authentic to be considered authoritative evidence of a transaction or event; records are authentic if they are created or sent by the agent claiming to have created or sent it.*

An authentic e-record is what it purports to be. The e-records are properly issued by an authorized regulated user or regulated entity.

Where an electronic system generates e-records, corresponding management measures and technical means should be adopted to ensure the authenticity of the information generated.

The expected regulated user performs the issuance of authentic e-records. This user must have a unique combination of user identification and password.

The e-records must remain unaltered while in transit. An authentic e-record is also gained after sending the e-record protected by any cryptographic based tools such as hashing, Virtual Private Network (VPN), Secure Sockets Layer (SSL), and so on.

As an example, the SSL protocol establishes an encrypted link between a server and a regulated user, typically a web server and a browser, or a mail server and a mail client. By authenticating a server, the person is assured of communication with the correct site. SSL also signs the transmitted e-records, so the person is assured that the e-records have not been changed in transit.

The risks that should be considered when checking the completeness and accuracy of e-records are [10]:

- Is original data (including the original data format) available for checking
- Are there any periods when data is not audit trailed?
- Does the data reviewer have visibility and access to all data generated?

- Does the data reviewer have visibility and access to all processing of data?

Requirement 15 - *Once a record has been captured into a records system, all events and actions related to the record by person entities and non-person entities must be documented on an ongoing basis.*

For electronic systems performing operations covered by the medicines' manufacturing practices regulations the way documenting modifications via audit trails. The items included in the audit trail should be relevant to reconstruct the generation, modification and deletion of the user management- and system settings.

An audit trail is another e-records that the integrity must be a safeguard. User access rights must be restricted to the audit trails to prevent amendments and switch off the audit trail. The access to the audit trails is limited to review and/or print only. The timestamp to the audit trails must be reliable.

Requirement 16 - *All records must be associated with the approved records schedules that pertain to each record.*

The requirements for retention of e-records and documents do not differ from paper documents per the companies Retention Schedule and applicable GxP regulations. It should ensure that electronic signatures applied to e-records are valid for the entire storage period for documents.

After the e-records are inactive and transferred to the retention environment for subsequent safekeeping and preservation, the e-records are logically categorized based on the planned, expected retention time for purging.

In addition to the e-records, audit trails, backups, paper related records and so on, associated with the e-records to be purged are purged as well.

From a legal perspective, it is important to remember that record handling programs include defined provisions to temporarily suspend the execution of the purge process when records are part of a legal discovery process during pending litigation.

REFERENCES

[1] MHRA, "*GxP Data Integrity Guidance and Definitions*," March 2018.
[2] Computerised systems. In: The rules governing medicinal products in the European Union. Volume 4: Good manufacturing practice (GMP) guidelines: Annex 11, June 2011.
[3] EMA, "*Guidance on good manufacturing practice and good distribution practice: Questions and answers, Data Integrity*," 2016.
[4] EMA, "*Guidance on good manufacturing practice and good distribution practice: Questions and answers, Data Integrity*," 2016.
[5] López, O., "*Trustworthy Computer Systems*" in Pharmaceutical and Medical Devices Regulation Operations, López, O., Eds (CRC Press, Boca Raton, FL, 1st ed., 2017), pp. 101-119.
[6] WHO, Technical Report Series No. 937, Annex 4. Appendix 5, "*Validation of computerized systems*", 2006.
[7] ISO 9241-210:2010, "*Ergonomics of human-system interaction - Part 210: Human-centered design for interactive systems*."
[8] 21 CFR Part 11. Title 21 Code of Federal Regulations Part 11 (21 CFR Part 11).
[9] López, O., "*Technologies Supporting Integrity of E-records*," in Pharmaceutical and Medical Devices Manufacturing Computer Systems Validation, López, O., Eds. (Routledge/Productivity Press, New York, NY, 1st ed., 2018), pp. 141-162
[10] EMA, "*Guidance on good manufacturing practice and good distribution practice: Questions and answers, Data Integrity*," 2016.

Chapter 9

E-RECORDS MAINTENANCE AND USE

INTRODUCTION

The e-records maintenance and use are the processes of managing e-records through their Active and Inactive phases. These managing e-records include processing, reviewing, analyzing, reporting, transferring, storing, transforming, migrating, archiving, and retrieving, so the e-records remain usable. Digital preservation is vital for e-records.

This chapter discusses the requirements associated with the e-records lifecycle during the maintenance and use activities.

The maintenance and use of e-records controls are contingent on the e-records phase state, Active or Inactive. E-records in the period of creation cannot be used nor maintained. Figure 3.1, E-records Lifecycle, provides a pictorial view of the Active and Inactive Phases, and Period of creation.

Active Phase

After the data is transformed and the corresponding built-in checks performed, there is a commitment to use the data. The data to be used is stored in the processing environment.

The data is stored in defined fields, becoming raw data (e.g., structured data). The raw data is used for their intended purposes as representing the activities they stand for. The raw data can be edited from the time it is saved in an electronic storage device through to final disposition [1]. When data "processability" is extended into the inactive phase, access and administration will also need to be extended ensuring controlled management of the modification to e-records.

The Active Phase encompasses e-records that are kept and accessed for their intended purpose. Activities associated with the Active Phase are e-records storage, access, transforming, modifying, periodically reviewing, analyzing, reporting, migrating, archiving, retaining, backing up, and restoring.

In addition to the audit trail functionality during the Active Phase, change management may represent governance that controls editing or modifying the e-records.

Resulting from the criticality of the raw data, periodically, raw data within the e-records may be cleansed to correct inconsistent values after using the data. This activity must be suitably managed using procedural control and documented (e.g., audit trail).

The three key CGMP controls to e-records in storage compliant with e-records integrity are:

- the modifications to CGMP e-records must be recorded at the time of modifying the e-records
- periodic complete backups [2] must be performed
- security controls must be established for all electronic storage devices and networks as a means of ensuring e-records protections

Inactive Phase

The Inactive Phase starts after the e-records in scope are inactive, superseded, replaced, and withdrawn. The e-records in scope are ingested [3].

When acquiring or developing the electronic archive, it is expected that consideration must be given to the long-term retention schedule requirements for these e-records, particularly concerning accessibility, readability, traceability and possibly any future processing needs through to final disposition.

Technical and functional requirement specifications for such electronic archives should include long-term storage, preservation, management and retrieval of their e-records. The requirements should consist of all the issues described in this section to ensure that e-records from these electronic archives can be archived in a manner that is compliant with all applicable requirements and industry best practices.

The key activities associated with maintaining inactive e-records are store, access, periodically reviewing, reporting, transferring, retaining, backing up, and restoring.

Three key requirements to maintain inactive CGMP e-records are:

- the archiving process must include verification that all e-records and associated metadata are not altered in value and/or meaning during the migration process
- archived e-records need to be verified periodically for accessibility, readability, integrity, and the state of security
- periodic complete and exact backups, secure from alteration, unintentional erasures, or loss

Maintenance and use are elements of the NIST stages of storage and processing.

E-Records Maintenance and Use Requirements

The following e-records maintenance and use requirements keep the e-records integrity as part of the lifecycle to the e-records.

Requirement 17 *- E-records must be managed in a manner that supports searching in response to information requests.*

Access to e-records, including searches, shall be limited to regulated users with a business need to access the associated e-records.

Access to the e-records shall be approved by the e-records owner or documented delegate before access is granted. All training shall be completed before granting access to trainees. A check shall be performed at the time of granting access to a new role whether the user has rights that allow a conflict of interest (segregation of role functions) [4].

Requirement 18 *- Access rights and permission rules for e-records should be adjusted to coincide with changes to the regulatory environment, to business activities, or the structure of the organization.*

Regulated users of electronic systems shall only have access to functionality within the system as required by their job role. User roles and responsibilities shall be pre-determined and documented in controlled documentation [4].

Requirement 19 *- Access rights and permission rules for e-records should be based on the function, activity, or business process related to the e-records. This allows for changes to be made to the organization without affecting the access and permission rules.*

The regulated user must exercise appropriate controls to assure that changes to CGMP e-records can be made only by authorized personnel 211.68(b)).

User access controls should ensure strict segregation of duties. The regulated user access rights and permissions align with personnel responsibilities [4].

Typically, users with elevated access rights (e.g., admin) should not conduct regular work tasks on the system.

To assist in controlling access, manufacturers must establish and implement a method for documenting authorized personnel's access privileges for each CGMP electronic system in use [4].

Requirement 20 - *Any actions changing the level of access, altering the e-record, or changing the location of the e-record must be documented and tracked into an audit log.*

As part of altering the e-record, audit trails refer to a journal, paper-based or computer-based, or version control that can trace the e-records alterations to the e-records.

Computer-generated and time-stamped electronic audits trails are preferred for tracking changes to electronic source e-records.

For regulated entities expectations on audit trails, refer to Requirement #14.

Related to changes in the location of the e-records, the repository for electronic e-records can be transferred because of servers or storage equipment replacement or upgrades, the retirement of electronic systems, website consolidation, server maintenance, and data centre relocation [4]. It is a consideration for any system implementation, upgrade, or consolidation.

Lastly, the creation, change, and cancellation of access levels must be recorded (EU Annex 11 p12.3) [5].

Instead of an audit trail, the changes in the e-records and changes to the access levels can be traced via a system log.

Requirement 21 - *The regulated entity must have e-records of a sustainability plan to maintain e-records over time.*

In this context, a sustainability plan is a roadmap to maintaining the quality of the e-records until the final disposal of the e-records.

The procedural controls to handling e-records during the Maintenance and Use Activities include system setup, installation, deployment and use, validation and functionality testing, data collection and handling, system maintenance, system security measures, security settings, security user's profiles, change control, e-record backup, recovery, contingency planning and decommissioning.

These procedural controls ensure that data is stored, archived, or disposed of safely and securely during and after the decommissioning of the electronic system.

Complementing the above procedural controls are the e-records management process. During the Maintenance and Use Activities the e-records management procedure must cover:

- Data modification
  - Ensure that the systems are designed to permit data changes in such a way that the e-records changes are documented and that there is no physical deletion of entered e-records (e.g., maintain an audit trail, data trail, edit trail) and associated metadata (e.g., data that describe the context, content and structure of the data).
  - Maintain a list of the users who are authorized to make e-records changes.
- Data review
  - Verification of data.
  - Traceability to raw data.
  - Changes to critical data traceable (analysis results, method parameters). The data traceability review should include the setup conditions used to generate the e-record or associated data.
  - What manual activities have been performed by whom and when?
  - If unprocessed raw data are not printed, the review must also include an electronic system to check for any user manipulation of data.
- Data Security - User access
  - Segregation of duty (analysis, review, admin tasks)

    - Analyst and reviewer must not have administrator rights.
    - Different personalized accounts for analysis and administration with additional mitigating controls (e.g., review of user access log) if recommended solution not possible for organizational reasons – controls need to be defined in a procedure.

- Data availability
  - Procedures should be in place to ensure that essential information remains complete and retrievable throughout the specified retention period.
    - Backup and restore
    - Disaster Recovery
    - Archival
  - Restore and Recovery procedures need to be tested to ensure technical controls do not compromise e-records integrity.
  - Restore and Recovery Procedures must require an appropriate authorization mechanism to prevent misuse.

Data quality is discussed in Chapter 15. The quality attributes must be preserved until the final disposal of the e-records.

Requirement 22 - *Ensuring usability of e-records means determining if the retention period for any e-records is longer than the life of the system where they are currently stored.*

E-records usability measures how well a specific regulated user in a specific context can use the e-records to achieve a defined goal effectively, efficiently and satisfactorily.

As the extended maintainability of the software and/or infrastructure technology obsolesce, e-records may be transferred to the retention environment while waiting for the completion of the retention period. This environment is used for the safekeeping and preservation of e-records.

Within this retention environment, e-records may take on a different form that would preserve their utility as informational objects without the need for original processing tools. In these environments, e-record access and use may require software and hardware different from those used for creation. Wherever retention environment is designed around the use of original processing tools to access stored e-records, additional controls may be required to secure the integrity of information from modification when using original creation tools for access. E-records that are transformed and placed in the retention environment, other than the environment used for original creation, should are to preserve the integrity of the source e-record and protection mechanisms used to prevent informational loss and/or corruption.

Should e-records require modifications in the retention environment, mechanisms must be engineered to enforce change documentation to preserve an audit trail of change or replacement history that includes also e-record removal [6]. These changes to records were recorded via an audit trail. These audit trails shall be retained at least if the e-record to which they pertain.

In any case, e-records transferred to the retention environment must be verified without altering the value, meaning, accessibility, readability, and integrity. (EU Annex 11 p4.8 and p.17)

In addition, in processing or retention environments, secure controls must be in place to ensure the integrity of the e-record throughout the retention period [8].

Requirement 23 - *Ensuring usability of e-records includes converting e-records to usable formats and maintaining the link between the e-records and their metadata through the conversion process.*

In the context of e-records usability and the regulated user, e-records can be converted in a different format and schema to satisfy the usability requirements.

If this is the case, during the conversion, it must be involved verifications to the converted e-records to demonstrate that the e-records are not altered in value and meaning.

The context and meaning of an e-record are contained in the metadata [9]. The metadata is linked to the respective e-record, and it is another e-record subject to all applicable e-records integrity controls. One of the e-records controls is that the link between the metadata and its e-records and not be removed.

Requirement 24 - *Ensuring usability of e-records includes ensuring that migration of e-records addresses non-active electronic e-records stored off-line.*

Data transfer/migration is the process of moving e-records and associated metadata between repositories for e-records or electronic systems. Data transfer/migration where required may change the data format for making it usable or visible on an alternative electronic system. (Russia)

There must be procedural control to manage the e-records transfer/migration. It should include a rationale and be robustly designed and to ensure that data integrity is maintained during the transfer/migration process.

The procedural control to manage transfer/migration must include instructions on how data will be migrated to new formats, operating systems, and so on so that e-records are readable throughout their entire lifecycles. Include in your migration planning provisions for transferring permanent e-records in the cloud to the regulated entity [9].

The transfer/migration of e-records between repositories for e-records requires specific planning, designing, verification, and testing. and control.

Careful consideration should be given to understanding the data format and the potential for alteration at each data generation, transfer and subsequent storage [10]. The Data Process Design related documentation, refer to Chapter 3, is the document in which data analysis is performed to obtain the e-records content, consistency, and structure.

Based on Figure 3.1, E-records Lifecycle, the active and inactive e-records must be migrated.

At the end of the transfer/migration, a verification and/or testing must be executed to demonstrate that the values of the e-records were not altered in the meaning, accessibility, readability, and integrity. (EU Annex 11 p4.8 and p.17)

The above verification/testing authenticates the completeness and accuracy of the transferred/migrated e-records. These verifications may use a statistically relevant sample [11].

Requirement 25 - *Ensuring usability of e-records includes carrying out system upgrades of hardware and software while maintaining the functionality and integrity of the e-records created in them.*

If modifications are to be performed to the processing and/or retention environments, then the ability to retrieve the e-record(s) should be ensured and tested. (EU Annex 11 p.17 [5])

Requirement 26 - *If their cloud provider discontinues services, the regulated user must continue to meet their e-records management responsibilities by migrating the e-records to another system or repository.*

E-records managed by a cloud service provider as agreed with the regulated entity, the contract giver, must comply with the migration of e-records. The responsibilities of the contract giver and the service provider should be clarified [12].

The responsibilities of all parties are written in a service level agreement (SLA). (EU Annex 11 p3.1 (50), including the discontinuing of the services by the cloud provider.

The SLA must also contain the monitoring and evaluation of cloud service providers by using contractual requirements relating to the management of e-records as evaluation criteria.

The SLA explains general actions regarding the migration of CGMP e-records. There must be a plan associated with the migration.

E-records migration is one of those activities addressed in the SLA. The e-records migration is the process of transferring e-records between storage types, formats, or computer systems. It is a key consideration for any system implementation, upgrade, or consolidation.

E-records automated migration is usually performed programmatically, freeing human resources from tedious tasks. E-records migration occurs for a variety of reasons, including server or storage equipment replacements or upgrades; retirement of computer systems; website consolidation; server maintenance; and data centre relocation [4].

The migration process must be well documented. Before any e-record can be migrated from one system to another, it is essential to identify differences between systems and how they might affect how reliably the migrated e-record can preserve and present information.

Changes in factors that affect how reliably an e-record can preserve and present information might not always be readily apparent. Examples of such changes include, but are not limited to, the following:

- moving from one type of record storage media to a different one
- installing a new version of an application or operating system software program
- moving from one electronic file format to another

Verification must be performed after concluding the migration process to ensure that the original e-records have not been altered or deleted from the electronic copy of the e-records. The verification should include corroboration that e-records are not changed in value, meaning, structure, context and links (e.g., audit trails, metadata) and/or meaning during this migration process.

Accessibility and readability verifications of the migrated e-records are also applicable after the migration of e-records.

In addition to the above verifications, migration testing should be performed long before the migration is complete. Testing must be performed throughout the migration process to catch errors and problems while still fixable. As soon as the migration process is complete, a team of data SMEs must perform a more comprehensive set of tests to assess and accept the new system before the users start using the migrated data set.

The migrated set of e-records must be assessed to ensure a high level of quality once the new repository becomes available to current and future users. The e-records quality assessment process should involve the removal of duplicate content and all files that are not relevant to current or future business processes and, if applicable, the creation of a master data file.

When system-level software is used to make an identical copy of an e-record, the system level software typically has a built-in error checking mechanism to help ensure that the copy is, in fact, a true copy.

Senior management is accountable for implementing systems and procedures, such as migrating e-records, minimizing the potential risk to data integrity [13] of e-records when cloud service provider discontinues services.

Requirement 27 - *The system receiving the migrated records must have appropriate security and records management controls in place to manage the records throughout the entire lifecycle, including preventing unauthorized access or disposal of records.*

In the situation referenced in Requirement #25, the service provider discontinues the service provided to the contract giver and the e-records stored in the cloud service provider need to be migrated to a new repository.

In this new setting, the e-records handling function must ensure that the e-records are safe and secure during and after the decommissioning of the electronic system.

As a function related to security, the e-records management controls preserve the e-records exactly as captured and created, and auditable to affirm reliability.

The records management controls include logical protections, stamped audit trail, records handling [14], archival and retrieval of records.

Requirement 28 - *Regulated companies must periodically review their e-records schedules to determine if changes to their use of technology affect the value of the records in question.*

Regulated e-records generated by electronic systems shall be retained in accordance, as a minimum, with the applicable regulatory requirements. In addition, regulated companies may have additional e-records retention schedules. Legal hold notices may increment the retention schedule. The e-records retention schedules also apply to corresponding audit trail entries and metadata.

Any changes to the computer system infrastructure (e.g., the repository for e-records), system software (e.g., operating system version, middle software), and/or application software managing the e-records must only be made in a controlled manner per a defined procedural control (EU Annex 11 p10 [5]).

Verification [15] to the e-records must be performed to evaluate the integrity, accessibility, retrievability, and legibility that will be impacted by the changes to the computer system infrastructure, system software, and/or application software.

Requirements 29 - *Records must be managed to support the export of e-records to facilitate access processing.*

To export is to convert a file into another format than the one it is currently in.

This exportation of e-records requires specific planned testing and controls [16]. As part of the exportation process, the validation process should include verifications that data are not altered in value and/or meaning (EU Annex 11 p 4.8 [5]).

The same principle is applicable when the exportation is between systems.

Requirement 30 - *The regulated entity must continuously review their records schedules to determine if changes to their business processes affect the value of the records in question.*

E-records and metadata should be retained for the periods specified in the associated predicate regulation. Disposition actions specified in the predicate regulations must be implemented.

The following are some of the possible changes to business processes that may affect the value of the records schedules.

- If a regulated entity needs to deviate from retention periods
- If a regulated entity needs to modify the description of e-records because the informational content of the records and/or the function documented by the records changes
- If the regulated entity decides to change the scope of the records, schedule items to include a greater or lesser aggregation of records

Requirement 31 - *Regulated entities should have the ability to configure workflows based on an organization's business process rules and transactional data, without custom programming.*

A CGMP workflow is a software application that automates, to at least some degree, a CGMP process. It is validated using an SLC. The extent of validation studies should be proportionate with the intended use and associated risk [17].

The requirement prefers configurable workflows instead of bespoke software workflows.

Configurable workflows are easiest to implement, validate, and maintain than bespoke software workflows.

Requirement 32 *- The repository of e-records should allow users to perform a full-text search of a record's content.*

A full-text search refers to methods for searching a collection of e-records in a full-text database and is a more advanced way to search a database. Full-text search is distinguished from searches based on metadata or parts of the original texts represented in databases.

It quickly finds all instances of a term (word) in a table without having to scan rows and know which column a term is stored in. Full-text search works by using text indexes.

The application providing access to the repository of e-records must allow the regulated users with authorization to access the e-records to perform a full-text search of a record's content.

Requirement 33 *- The repository of e-records must allow the regulated entity to identify and categorize any e-records considered critical.*

The regulated data should be categorized based on a criticality assessment. The criticality of data is based on the impact of the data on final product quality. Critical data is data with a high risk to product quality or patient safety [18].

The application providing access to the repository of e-records must have the functionality to allow regulated users with access to the e-records to search data and categorize e-records as critical.

REFERENCES

[1] Disposition - Range of processes associated with implementing records retention or destruction.
[2] A complete backup includes all relevant raw GxP data, metadata and audit trail data.

[3] Ingestion - The process that accepts electronic records for archiving. (SAG, "*A Guide to Archiving of Electronic Records*," February 2014).

[4] CEFIC, "*Practical Risk-based Guide for Managing Data Integrity*," March 2019 (Rev 1).

[5] EudraLex, The Rules Governing Medicinal Products in the European Union, Volume 4, "*EU Guidelines to Good Manufacturing Practice, Medicinal Products for Human and Veterinary Use Part 1, Annex 11 - Computerized Systems*," June 2011.

[6] ISPE/PDA, "*Good Practice and Compliance for Electronic Records and Signatures. Part 1 Good Electronic Records Management (GERM)*". July 2002.

[7] *EudraLex, The Rules Governing Medicinal Products in the European Union,* Volume 4, Good Manufacturing Practice Medicinal Products for Human and Veterinary Use, Chapter 4: Documentation, June 2011.

[8] Metadata are data that describe the attributes of other data and provide context and meaning. (CEFIC)

[9] Federal Records Management, NARA Bulletin 2010-05: *Guidance on Managing Records in Cloud Computing Environments*, September 2010.

[10] MHRA. (March 2018). "'*GxP' Data Integrity Guidance and Definitions*."

[11] CEFIC, "*Practical risk-based guide for managing data integrity*," March 2019 (Version 1)

[12] National Medical Products Association (NMPA (former CFDA)), "*Drug Data Management Practices Guidance*," December 2020.

[13] MHRA. (March 2018). "*'GxP' Data Integrity Guidance and Definitions.*"

[14] Data Handling - The process of ensuring that data is stored, archived, or disposed of safely and securely during the data lifecycle.

[15] Verification - The process of determining whether the products of a given phase of the SLC fulfil the requirements established during the previous phase.

[16] WHO. (October 2019). *Guideline on Data Integrity* (QAS/19.819 Draft)

[17] US FDA, "*Data Integrity and Compliance with Drug CGMP - Questions & Answers - Guidance for industry*," December 2018.

[18] *ISPE GAMP COP Annex 11 – Interpretation, Pharmaceutical Engineering*, July/August 2011.

Chapter 10

E-RECORDS DISPOSAL

INTRODUCTION

E-records disposal is the process of setting e-records scheduled for discard. The requirements for the disposal of e-records and electronic documents do not differ from paper documents.

E-records that meet the retention requirements are disposed of in accordance, as an example, to the NIST Special Publication 800-88 [1]. E-records scheduled for destruction must be disposed of in a manner that ensures protection of any privacy, proprietary, or company information.

The documented e-records disposal process should be in place to ensure that the correct original records or true copies are disposed of after the defined retention period. The system should ensure that current records are not destroyed by accident and that historical records do not inadvertently make their way back into the current record stream [2].

In addition to the e-records, the content, attributes, and audit trails of each e-records are discarded as well [3].

A record/register should be available to demonstrate appropriate and timely archiving or destruction of retired records per local policies [2].

E-RECORDS DISPOSAL REQUIREMENTS

The following e-records disposal requirements keep the media holding the e-records sanitized [4].

Requirement 34 - *E-records must be disposed of in a manner that protects any sensitive, proprietary, or company information. Any e-recording media previously used for e-records containing sensitive, proprietary, or company information must not be reused if the previously recorded information can be compromised in any way by the reuse of the media.*

Suppose the e-records are restricted because they contain sensitive, proprietary, or company information and are scheduled for destruction. If this is the case, e-records must be disposed of in a manner that ensures the protection of any sensitive, proprietary, or company information.

The magnetic recording media previously used for e-records containing sensitive, proprietary, or company information must not be reused if the previously recorded information can be compromised in any way by the reuse of the media.

Requirement 35 - *Regulated entity must control any proposed deletion of e-records according to existing e-records retention schedules.*

The application of approved physical deletion schedules is mandatory. E-records must be retained as specified by the predicate regulation.

The objective of the procedural and technological controls is to avoid the erasure of e-records in an unauthorized manner [5].

Logical security is the most effective control to avoid the deletion of e-records in an unauthorized manner. It includes all precautions to e-records against unauthorized deletion of e-records.

Network-specific security procedures (network security and database server) control the access to individual computer system platforms. Access to these devices should be maintained (logical security).

The access rights allowing the disposal of e-records should be controlled and restricted to limited persons.

Unnecessary networked services should be disabled and secured. Like most operating systems and complex applications, database software provides some services that allow remote system management, distributed processing, and other network-related functions. In many cases, those services are enabled by default and are often 'protected' using either no password or a vendor-supplied default password.

E-records security includes integrity, reliability and availability of these e-records. During validation of a database or inclusive system, consideration should be given to [6]:

- implementing procedures and mechanisms to ensure data security (e.g., user access to the e-records and user permissions to perform activities in the database) and keeping the meaning and logical arrangement of data.
- load-testing, considering future growth of the database and tools to monitor the saturation of the database.
- precautions for necessary migration of data (EU Annex 11 p17 [7]) at the end of the system's lifecycle.

Complete back-ups provide the ability to protect the e-records from system failure, erasure and the ability to recover the e-records.

For the above reasons, e-records must be regularly and progressively backed up, and the backup retained at a remote and secure location. For recovery, the backup must be complete [8].

The procedural controls establishing the backup process must be in place for ensuring the integrity of backups (secure storage location, adequately separated from the primary storage location, and error-free). This backup may be part of a more general disaster recovery plan.

Following changes to the system and/or backup utility, change control should ensure the availability and integrity of the backup files and stored data by comparing backup data and the original files backed up on a trial basis.

The integrity and accuracy of backup data and the ability to restore the data should be checked during validation and monitored periodically.

The frequency of back-ups depends on data criticality, amount of stored data and frequency of data generation.

Requirement 36 - *All e-records must be covered by an approved disposition authority.*

The regulatory requirements cover the application of approved schedules. Regulated companies may have extended disposition schedules mandatory, such as legal discovery process during pending litigation or a deviation relayed investigation.

During the E-records Final Disposition Phase, those company e-records, meeting the approved retention time, are tagged to discard and removed according to an approved procedure. The purged e-record information typically includes content, metadata, audit trails, and any pointers to the e-record and connections to related e-records. The e-record must be eliminated as well in the retention environment. Refer to Chapter 3.

Where an e-record is deleted before meeting its approved retention schedule, an audit trail of the deletion is good practice until the end of the agreed retention period.

Current good practice also includes, as part of a company's e-records handling program, a periodic verification to revisit the approved retention of periods of specific e-records as business, regulatory or legal requirements change.

Requirement 37 - *If a suspend-disposition regulated authority or legal hold is issued, the disposition of approved e-records must cease immediately. The approved e-records will remain suspended until a* *revocation order lifts the regulated authority. Once the authority is lifted, the disposition of approved e-records can continue.*

A regulated entity must extend the e-records retention periods when a legal hold is effective.

An example of extending the disposition is raw data during failure investigations under CAPA.

A procedural control must control the process when a suspend-disposition regulated authority or legal hold is issued,

Requirement 38 - *Regulated entities may retain e-records approved for physical deletion beyond the period outlined in the e-records schedule if the e-records in question pertain to a court order, executive order, law, or approved business justification*

Regulated entities must not retain e-records whose physical deletion after a specified period is required by the regulatory authority.

Once the special circumstances that require extended e-records have elapsed, the regulated entity must physically delete the e-records per the approved disposition instructions.

Such extension can come as outlined in Requirement #36.

Requirement 39 - *Once the circumstances about the extended retention of e-records are no longer applicable, the regulated entity must destroy the e-records per the e-records schedule.*

Secure controls must be in place to ensure the e-records integrity of the e-record throughout the whole retention period [9]. This applies to corresponding audit trail entries and metadata as well.

Disposition actions specified in the predicate regulations must be implemented. These are standard.

For example, batch documentation must be kept for one year after the expiry of the batch to which it relates or at least five years after certification of the batch by the Qualified Person [10], whichever is the longer [11].

Legal hold notices may increment the retention schedule. The legal hold notices are resolved by legal authorities, not by the associated predicate regulation.

Periodically, the legal holds must be reviewed to ensure the impact on the legal hold linked e-records and avoid inadvertent loss of e-records due to erasing e-records already expired by the associated predicate rule with an indefinite legal hold.

To erase regulated e-records, the legal hold and the regulatory disposition must be expired.

REFERENCES

[1] NIST, "*Guidelines for Media Sanitization, SP 800-88*", Revision 1, December 2014.

[2] MHRA, "*GxP Data Integrity Guidance and Defin*itions," March 2018.

[3] ISPE/PDA, "*Good Practice and Compliance for Electronic Records and Signatures. Part 1 Good Electronic Records Management (GERM)*". July 2002.

[4] In the context of this book sanitization refers to a process that renders access to target data on the media useless for a given level of effort. (NIST SP 800-88)

[5] ISO 15489-1:2016(E) - *Records Management.*

[6] European Medicines Agency (EMA) - GMP/GDP compliance – "*Questions and answers: Good manufacturing practice: Annex 11 Computerised Systems Question 4*," http://www.ema.europa.eu/ema/index.jsp?curl=pages/regulation/q_and_a/q_and_a_detail_000027.jsp&mid=WC0b01ac05800296ca#section9

[7] EudraLex, The Rules Governing Medicinal Products in the European Union, Volume 4, "*EU Guidelines to Good Manufacturing Practice, Medicinal Products for Human and*

Veterinary Use Part 1, Annex 11 - Computerized Systems," June 2011.

[8] A complete backup includes all relevant raw GxP data, metadata and audit trail data.

[9] MHRA. (March 2018). *'GxP' Data Integrity Guidance and Definitions*

[10] Qualified person - Persons qualified to prescribe medicinal products must be able to carry out these functions objectively without being influenced by direct or indirect financial inducements.

[11] *EudraLex, The Rules Governing Medicinal Products in the European Union,* Volume 4, Good Manufacturing Practice Medicinal Products for Human and Veterinary Use, Chapter 4: Documentation, June 2011.

Chapter 11

E-RECORDS TRANSFER

INTRODUCTION

The E-records transfer is the process of moving e-records and metadata between storage media types or electronic systems via an interface [1].

The general regulatory requirements to transfer e-records involve, among other things, that the e-records are readily available as necessary to be disposed of safely and securely during the retention period. This safe and secure disposal of e-records includes generating accurate and complete copies of e-records suitable for inspection, review, and copying by, the regulatory entities [2].

In general, the worldwide regulatory authorities will consider electronic copies of e-records accurate and complete if they convey all the information and revisions as in the original e-records.

The typical e-records transfer can be between different e-records storage types, formats, or computer systems.

Where e-records are exchanged between two or more systems, the ease of e-records transfer can be facilitated using a standard exchange format [3].

E-records migration is considered e-records transfer as well.

An additional form of e-records transfer is the backups.

E-records transfer/migration procedures should include a rationale and be robustly designed, and the process validated to ensure that e-records integrity is maintained during the e-records lifecycle. Careful consideration should be given to understanding the e-records format and the potential for alteration at each stage of e-records generation, transfer and subsequent storage.

The E-records transfer is an element of the NIST data transmission.

E-Records Transfer Controls While in Transit [4]

For various reasons, e-records may be moved between systems via a computer interface. The controls associated with moving e-records via the interface must ensure that the moved e-records have remained unaltered during the transit via an interface.

Interfaces between electronic systems present e-records integrity risk whereby e-records may be inadvertently lost, amended or transcribed incorrectly during the transfer process [5].

Verification methods may include the use of:

- secure transfer
- encryption
- checksums

During the set-up and qualification, the controls should deliver confidence that:

- the e-records residing at the receiving system are the precise representation of the e-records generated at the source system.
- no regulated users can manipulate e-records during the transferring process.

The following are the controls associated with e-records while in transit.

Qualification of Computer Infrastructure [6]

After computer infrastructure is designed or selected and installed, it should be evaluated and tested to verify that it can operate satisfactorily within the operating limits required by the software.

Qualification [7] of the computer infrastructure includes:

- service design.
- service delivery, including installation and evaluation of the system.
- change control, maintenance and calibration, security, contingency planning, training, performance monitoring and periodic re-evaluation.

The computer infrastructure must conform to the regulated entity established standards through a planned verification process building upon acknowledged good IT practices. Once in conformance, this state must be maintained by established processes and QA controls, the effectiveness of which must be periodically verified [8].

Build-in Checks

Computer systems exchanging e-records electronically with other systems should include, if technically feasible, appropriate built-in checks for the correct computer inputs and outputs (I/Os).

Built-in Checks (EU Annex 11 p5, US FDA 211.68(b), and US FDA CPG 7132a.07 Computerized Drug Processing; Input/Output Checking [9]) include the correct and secure entry and processing of e-records ensuring the completeness of in transit e-record acquisition and the accurate and secure entry and processing of e-records, to minimize e-records integrity risks.

"*Why are built-in checks required for electronic interfaces if the interface has been validated? [10]* The question cannot be answered as such. The checks of data built in the interface are tested within validation. Changes in a system can be problematic if they concern data that is transferred via that interface." Besides, interfaces are mainly hardware infrastructure in nature. Equipment malfunction cannot work correctly due to hardware deterioration [11].

The accurate I/Os ensures the secure exchange of e-records between systems and correct inputs on the processing of e-records. These built-in checks maximize the mitigation associated with I/Os errors.

The impact on network-based technologies is that insufficient error checking at the transaction entry point can result in incorrect transaction processing and e-records integrity risks. Integrity can be lost when e-records are processed incorrectly or when incorrectly handled transactions due to errors or delayed processing.

The built-in check is the mechanism that can ensure the reliability of the e-records transmissions and the mutual trust between communicating parties.

The built-in check provides:

- shared node authentication to assure each node of the others' identity.
- transmission integrity to guard against improper information modification or destruction while in transit.
- transmission confidentiality to ensure that information in transit is not disclosed to unauthorized individuals, entities, or processes.

This built-in check mechanism can support application and machine credentials and user machines (user nodes).

Critical to secure information exchange is a method to guarantee receiving exactly what the sender intended between electronic systems interfaces at the point of transaction entry. For this case, it is suggested that a "checksum" be utilized to ensure file integrity [11]. A checksum or hash sum is a fixed-size datum computed from an arbitrary block of digital e-records to detect errors that may have been introduced during a file's transmission or storage. The integrity of the e-records can be checked at any later time by re-computing the checksum for the file and comparing it with the stored checksum value. If the checksum values do not match, the e-records were almost certainly altered (either intentionally or unintentionally).

The use of a checksum for transmitting files provides several benefits, including:

- The integrity of each file can be verified by comparing the checksum submitted with the file and the computed checksum calculated upon receipt.
- The checksum can be used to verify that the file has not been altered in the historical archive. It is particularly useful as files are migrated from one storage medium to another (e.g., when files are backed up to magnetic tape storage).

In addition to all the above controls, computer, network, and interfaces must be verified periodically to ensure correct communication between components [12]. Likewise, the computer logs provide information about interface errors.

Accuracy Checks

Accuracy Checks is described in the EU Annex 11 p6. The critical e-records entered manually by an authorized person into the electronic system require input verification to prevent incorrect e-records entry. The accuracy check intends to confirm an independent verification record to show that the e-records entered manually were entered accurately.

The independent e-records verification to the manually entered critical e-records can be performed by a second authorized person or an electronic system.

Critical e-records transferred between electronic systems or from an electronic system to paper, the verification of accuracy can be performed by a second person or, if the system is appropriately validated, by the electronic system itself.

There should be no difference between manual input by the user and the take-over of e-records from another system. In the same way, processing operations performed by the system should be checked by the system itself or by a second person, as appropriate.

The impact on network-based technologies is that insufficient error checking at the transaction entry point can result in incorrect transaction processing and e-records integrity risks. Integrity can be lost when e-records are processed incorrectly or when incorrectly handled transactions due to errors or delayed processing.

In the context of the electronic system check, verification is programmed into the background of the e-records entry and configured to ensure the accuracy of the e-records input. It could be specific checks on e-records format, ranges or values.

As the system automatically compares e-records on input with predefined limits, as an example, the user should be warned of potential errors when the e-records is entered manually or as an input from another electronic system. For security purposes, the validity of the source of e-records input may be determined.

Faulty e-records entry can trigger a chain of events that result in a serious production error and the possible distribution of an adulterated product. Thus, while increasingly sophisticated system safeguards and computer monitoring of essential equipment and programs help protect e-records, no automated system exists that can completely substitute for human oversight and supervision.

Contemporaneous Record

The evidence of actions, events or decisions shall be recorded immediately after the e-record is captured. The e-records shall serve as an accurate attestation of what was done, or what was decided and why [14, 15].

E-Records Transfer between Storage Types and/or Format

An E-records transfer is a process of transferring e-records between different e-records storage types, formats, or electronic systems [15]. The e-records residing at the receiving system represent the e-records generated at the sending system [16].

Interfaces should be assessed and addressed during the validation process to ensure the correct and complete transfer of e-records [5].

The e-records should not be altered during or after it is transferred to the worksheet or other application. There should be an audit trail for this process. Appropriate Quality procedures should be followed if the e-records transfer during the operation has not occurred correctly. Any changes in the middle layer software should be managed through appropriate Quality Management Systems [18].

Where conversion to the new e-records format of the new software is not possible, the old software should be maintained installed in one computer and available as a backup media to have the opportunity to read the archived e-records in case of an investigation [19].

As in e-records migration, e-records transfer procedural control should include a rationale and be robustly designed and validated to ensure that e-records integrity is maintained during the e-records lifecycle. Careful consideration should be given to understanding the e-records format and the potential for alteration at each stage of e-records generation, transfer and subsequent storage.

E-RECORDS MIGRATION [20]

E-records migration is moving stored e-records from one durable storage location to another. It may include changing the format of e-records, but not the content or meaning. The modification of the format may be performed to make it usable or visible on an alternative electronic system.

E-records migration is usually performed programmatically to achieve an automated migration, freeing up human resources from tedious tasks. E-records migration occurs for various reasons, including server or storage equipment replacements or upgrades; retirement of electronic systems; website consolidation; server maintenance; and e-records centre relocation.

Before any e-record can be migrated, it is essential to identify differences between systems and how they might affect how reliably the migrated e-record can preserve and present information. Besides, precautions should be taken for the end of lifecycle e-records migration.

Changes in factors that affect how reliably an e-record can preserve and present information might not always be readily apparent. Examples of such differences include, but are not limited to, the following:

- moving from one type of record storage media to a different one.
- installing a new version of an application or operating system software program.
- moving from one electronic file format to another.

Verification must be performed after concluding the migration process to ensure that the original e-records has not been altered in or deleted from the electronic copy of the e-records. The verification should include corroboration that e-records are not altered in value, meaning, structure, context and links (e.g., audit trails, metadata) and/or meaning during this migration process.

Accessibility and readability verifications of the migrated e-records are also applicable after the migration of e-records.

In addition to the above verifications, migration testing should be performed long before the migration is complete. Testing must be performed throughout the migration process to catch errors and problems while they're still fixable. As soon as the migration process is complete, a team of e-records SME must perform a more comprehensive set of tests to assess and accept the new system before the users start using the migrated e-records set.

The migrated set of e-records must be assessed to ensure a high level of quality once the new repository becomes available to current and future users. The e-records quality assessment process should involve the removal of duplicate content and all files that are not relevant to current or future business processes and, if applicable, the creation of a master e-records file.

When system-level software is used to make an identical copy of an e-record, the system level software typically has a built-in error checking mechanism to help ensure that the copy is, in fact, a true copy.

The challenges of migrating e-records are often underestimated, particularly regarding maintaining the whole meaning of the migrated records.

The migration process procedures shall include a rationale and be robustly designed and verified to ensure that e-records integrity is maintained during the e-records lifecycle [17].

E-Records Backups

A backup is a copy of current (editable) e-records, metadata, audit trails, e-signatures and associated links, and system configuration settings maintained for disaster recovery [18]. The items included in an audit trail should be relevant to permit the reconstruction of the process or activity.

These e-records must be protected by backup transfer on magnetic tape, microfilm, electronic discs, paper printouts or other means. The e-records must be readily available during the retention period.

US FDA 21 CFR Part 211.68 requires that exact and complete and that it is secure from alteration, inadvertent erasures, or loss shall be maintained.

These technological controls provide the ability to keep the e-records from system failure and recover the e-records. Besides, backups shall be performed for recovery issues and as part of the backout plan before any system upgrade or maintenance activity.

For the above reasons, e-records must be regularly and progressively backed up, and a copy of the backup retained at a remote and secure location. The backup and copies must also have the same appropriate controls to prohibit unauthorized access to, changes to and deletion of e-records or their alteration [16].

A procedural control establishes that the backup process must be in place to ensure the integrity of backups (secure storage location, adequately separated from the primary storage location, and error-free). This backup may be an element of a disaster recovery plan.

Following changes to the system and/or backup utility, change control should confirm the availability and integrity of the backup files and stored e-records by comparing backup e-records and the original files backed up on a trial basis.

The integrity and accuracy of backup e-records and the ability to restore the e-records should be checked during validation and monitored periodically.

The frequency of backups depends on the criticality of the e-records, number of stored e-records and frequency of e-records generation.

Note that backup differs from archival copies of electronic records are typically only temporarily stored for disaster recovery and may be periodically overwritten. Such temporary backup copies should not be relied upon as an archival mechanism [21].

REFERENCES

[1] An *interface is a shared boundary. To interact or communicate with another system component.* (ANSI/IEEE)

[2] 21 CFR Part 11.10(b)

[3] ISPE/PDA, "*Good Practice and Compliance for Electronic Records and Signatures. Part 1 Good Electronic Records Management (GERM)*". July 2002.

[4] López, O., "*Data Integrity in Pharmaceutical and Medical Devices Regulation Operations: Best Practices Guide to Electronic Records Compliance,*" CRC Press, Boca Ratón, Fl., 2017.

[5] PIC/S Pharmaceutical Inspection Convention. (July 2021). PIC_S PI 041-1, *Good Practice for Data Management and Integrity in Regulated GMPGDP Environments.*

[6] López, O. "*Computer Infrastructure Qualification for FDA Regulated Industries,*" PDA and DHI Publishing, LLC. 2006.

[7] WHO, Technical Report Series No. 937, Annex 4. Appendix 5, "*Validation of computerized systems*", Section 6.3, 2006.

[8] Cappucci, W.; Chris Clark, C.; Goossens, T.; Wyn, S., "*ISPE GAMP CoP Annex 11 Interpretation*", Pharmaceutical Engineering, July/August 2011.

[9] www.fda.gov/regulatory-information/search-fda-guidance-documents/cpg-sec-425400-computerized-drug-processing-inputoutput-checking

[10] Mangel, A., "Q&A on Annex 11," *GMP Journal*, Issue 8, April/May 2012.

[11] ICH, "*Electronic Standards for the Transfer of Regulatory Information*", June 2015, https://www.ich.org/page/multidisciplinary- guidelines.

[12] US FDA, "CPG Section 425.400 - Computerized Drug Processing; Input/Output Checking (CPG 7132a.07)," September 1987.

[13] Critical Data - data with high risk to product quality or patient safety. (ISPE GAMP COP Annex 11 – Interpretation, July/August 2011).

[14] WHO. (September 2015). "*Guide on Good Data and Record Management.*"

[15] MHRA. (March 2018). *'GxP' Data Integrity Guidance and Definitions'*.

[16] CEFIC, "Practical Risk-based Guide for Managing Data Integrity," March 2019 (Rev 1).

[17] (Russian) Federal State Institute of Drugs and Good Practices, "*Data Integrity & Computer System Validation*," (Draft) August 2018.

[18] MHRA. (March 2018). *'GxP' Data Integrity Guidance and Definitions'*.

[19] PI 041-1, "Good Practice for Data Management and Integrity in Regulated GMPGDP Environments," (PIC/S) July 2021.

[20] López, O., "Data *Integrity in Pharmaceutical and Medical Devices Regulation Operations: Best Practices Guide to Electronic Records Compliance,*" CRC Press, Boca Ratón, Fl., 2017.

[21] WHO, "*Annex 4 - Good chromatography practices*," in WHO Technical Report Series, no. 1025, 2020.

Chapter 12

METADATA

INTRODUCTION

A good metadata administration approach is the foundation for any serious data single-minded organization.

Metadata [1] is the data that provides information about other data. The term refers to information that gives context to data sets [2] and helps companies understand what they're looking at when they assess their numbers.

It provides the contextual information required to understand those data and reconstruct activities. Metadata is necessary to evaluate the meaning of data securely linked to the data and subject to adequate review. An information system can use metadata for three primary purposes: data management, data access and data analysis. Metadata enables retrievability across systems and usability across time. An e-record element provides meaning to e-record content, helps define the e-record structure, and ensures e-record integrity, usability, authenticity, and audibility. For this reason, metadata must be given the same degree of importance as the data it describes.

An audit trail is a form of metadata containing information associated with actions related to the creation, modification, or deletion of e-records.

An audit trail allows for securely recording lifecycle details such as creation, additions, omissions, or alterations in an e-record without obscuring or overwriting the original e-record. An audit trail facilitates e-records history reconstruction events, regardless of its medium, including the "who, what, when and why" [3].

Metadata is easily managed through a concept called a data dictionary [4], where for a given class of related data elements, data definitions are established and referenced for consistency. Many higher-end technologies have incorporated this concept in utilities supporting the construction and servicing of software databases. The idea can still be applied where the technology does not support a data dictionary. Still, human actions would require constructing and service the dictionary or encoding definitions within the source language. In either case, it is a good practice to define and preserve metadata as an essential part of data used in records, as it aids in the interpretation and meaning of data.

Where e-records are exchanged between two or more systems, can facilitate the ease of e-records transfer by using a standard exchange format. The portability of data between and across diverse computing environments adds another level to the concept of metadata. It is crucial to consider exchange standards utilized as that metadata used by technology to interpret and present data as information to the human user.

There may not be the capability to search across the unstructured data that has been captured. Until now, can perform searches across the metadata of that unstructured data.

The periodic e-records review is a process where the raw data and metadata are reviewed for their integrity in an individual data set.

Metadata for e-records should depict the following [5]:

- business context.
- dependencies and relationships among records and records systems.
- connections to legal and social contexts.
- relationships to agents who create, manage and use records.

Some records' metadata is derived or attributed when the e-record is created or captured and does not change. It is the point of capturing metadata for e-records.

Metadata about actions on the e-record and other events in the record's existence, including the participating agents, continue to accrue over time as the e-record is used and managed. It is process metadata for e-records.

As metadata accumulates over time, it collectively documents, amongst other things, a record's derivation.

The metadata of an e-record itself should be managed as an e-record. It should be protected from loss or unauthorized deletion and retained or destroyed following requirements identified as part of the retention of the associated e-record. Access to metadata should be controlled using authorized access and permissions rules.

The following aspects should be considered when determining risk and control measures related to metadata [6]:

- What metadata is associated with the e-record, ensuring e-record reliability?
- Does the e-record permit the reconstruction of the activity?
- Where is the metadata located? When metadata is stored in different file locations from raw data, the backup process should be carefully designed to ensure that all necessary data to reconstruct a record is included.
- Is it possible to recreate, amend or delete metadata?

E-Records Metadata Requirements

The following metadata requirements provide meaning to e-record content, helps to define the e-record structure, and ensures e-record integrity, usability, authenticity and audibility.

Requirement 40 - *Records systems [7] must define metadata to enable the identification and retrieval of records; associate records with changing business rules, policies, and mandates; associate records with agents, and their authorizations and rights with regards to the records; associate records with their business activities; track processes carried out on records.*

This requirement is self-explained.

It is essential to highlight that e-records that do not possess such metadata lack the characteristics of authoritative records.

Authoritative e-records are e-records that have the features of authenticity [8], reliability [9], integrity [10] and usability [11]. The authoritative e-record has evidence of business events or transactions and fully meet the requirements of the business [5].

Requirement 41 - *Metadata to manage records must be in one of six categories: (a) Identity - information identifying the record; (b) Description - information determining the nature of the record; (c) Use - information facilitating immediate and longer-term record use; (d) Event plan - information used to manage the record, such as disposition information; (e) Event history - information recording past events on the record and its metadata; (f) Relation - information describing the relationship between the record and other records.*

The identity metadata is the attributes of a record that characterize it as unique and distinguish it from other records. Examples of identity metadata include, among other elements, the names of the persons concurring in its creation; the date(s) and time(s) of issuing, creation and transmission; the matter or action in which it participates; the expression of its archival bond; the indication of any attachment(s); a digital signature; and the name of the person responsible for the business matter. Identity metadata is distinguished from integrity metadata "that accounts for the handling of records in digital systems from this point of creation to the end of permanent preservation.

The description metadata is information that represents the content and context of a resource that can be used to support understanding and discovery. Descriptive metadata often includes information about a resource's creator, its title and other identifiers, abstract or description of the content, keywords, date, form and genre, and other aspects that may help users determine if it is relevant to their queries.

Requirement 42 - *The metadata for a record must be protected from unauthorized deletion and must be retained or destroyed following the record's retention schedule.*

As in the parent record, all the e-records management requirements apply to metadata, including protecting e-records in storage (Chapter 8) and according to the retention schedule (Chapter 10).

Requirement 43 - *Once the record has been captured, the associated metadata must be fixed and kept as transactional evidence. The metadata includes a unique identifier, author, date of creation, and relationships with other records.*

The metadata repository shall be entirely outside the control and access of users, except for read-only access of this file. Each e-record in the metadata repository must be secure from subsequent unauthorized alteration (authority checks). The ability to change the metadata must be restricted to a minimum number of individuals and to duly authorize personal. Metadata should only be changeable by the following role: System Administrator with proper change control.

The metadata repository must be built using a unique identifier to trace the related e-record.

Requirement 44 - *Once the record has been captured, the associated metadata must be fixed and kept as transactional evidence. The metadata includes a unique identifier, author, date of creation, and relationships with other records.*

In a manufacturing environment, as an example, after the data is recorded and retained by an electronic storage device (e.g., Historian/SCADA storage, refer to Figure 3.2), the physical and logical controls to the e-records must be implemented and deployed. These controls include security, access authorization, backups, periodic reviews, stamped audit trails, metadata repository, built-in checks [12], and other relevant data handling controls. The PLC manages the alarms and the associated actions to the alarms. These alarm records are saved in the corresponding repository system at the storage device level.

Taking as an example the audit trails, the metadata includes the following fields:

- Data and time stamps of the action include the time zone reference.
- Identification of the person who has acted.
- The entry/value before the modification.
- The reason for the improvement. This entry would be manually entered.

The above information facilitates the reconstruction of the history of such events relating to the e-record.

Requirement 45 - *When migrating records, all metadata must be preserved and accompanied with the transfer.*

Because metadata provides meaning, context and definition to the associated e-records, it is essential that when e-records are transferred (Refer to Chapter 11), that the metadata associated with the e-records be preserved during any data manipulation process for migrating, reformatting or copying actions which support transfer activities. In e-records transfer, specific metadata may need to be transformed to retain context, structure, and knowledge preservation in the new computing environment.

Requirement 46 - *Transferred e-records must include the following metadata elements: File Name, Record ID, Title, Description, Creator, Creation Date, Rights. Metadata elements such as Coverage and Relation must also be provided if they apply to the records being transferred.*

The metadata elements below provide the minimum list of metadata terms necessary for describing e-records [13].

- File Name - The complete name of the computer file, including its extension (if present)
- Record ID - The unique identifier assigned by an agency or a records management system.
- Title - The name given to the record.
- Description - A narrative description of the content of the record, including abstracts for document-like objects or content descriptions for audio or video records.
- Creator - The regulated user or regulated company primarily responsible for the creation of the record
- Creation Date - The date that the file met the definition of a record. If a file (such as a case file, database or spreadsheet) holds multiple records created at different times, this element should note the date the file was created, and the span of dates recorded in the element Coverage.
- Rights - The classification allocated to the record indicating its official security status.
- Coverage - The geographic extent or scope of the content of the record.
- Relation - A related record that is either physically or logically required to form a complete record.

Requirement 47 - *Records can represent more than one business activity and therefore can be assigned to more than one record category.*

The connection between like records is designated within the Records Management Service by assignment of a record category – this implements the concept of the archival bond. The accumulation of records within a category set provides evidence of the manner of a business process or activity over time.

A record category is a graphic term that identifies the relationships between a record and other records resulting from the same business activity; one way of implementing archival bonds.

References

[1] ISPE/PDA, "*Good Practice and Compliance for Electronic Records and Signatures. Part 1 Good Electronic Records Management (GERM)*". July 2002.

[2] A data set is a collection of data. In the case of tabular data, a data set corresponds to one or more database tables. Every column of a table represents a variable, and each row corresponds to a given record of the data set in question. (Wikipedia)

[3] WHO. (October 2019). "*Guideline on Data Integrity*" (QAS/19.819 Draft)

[4] *Data Dictionary* - A data dictionary, or metadata repository, is a "centralized repository of information about data such as meaning, relationships to other data, origin, usage, and format". (*IBM Dictionary of Computing*)

[5] ISO 15489-1:2016(E), "*Information and documentation — Records management - Part 1: Concepts and principles*."

[6] EMA, "*EMA Questions and answers: Good manufacturing practice: Data integrity*," August 2016.

[7] A system of record (SOR) is an information storage and retrieval system (ISRS) that is the authoritative source for a data element in a system containing multiple sources of the same element. To ensure data integrity, there must be one, and only one record system for a given piece of information. (whatis.com)

[8] Authenticity - The property of being genuine and being able to be verified and trusted; confidence in the validity of a transmission, a message, or message originator. See authentication. (NIST Special Publication 800-18)

[9] Reliability - A reliable record is one whose contents can be trusted as a full and accurate representation of the transactions, activities, or facts to which they attest and can be depended upon during subsequent transactions or activities. (NARA)

[10] Integrity - The property that the data is complete and that has not been altered in an unauthorized manner. Data integrity covers data entry or collection, storage, transmission, and processing. (Note: Completeness is the property that all necessary parts of the entity in question are included)

[11] Usability - A useable record can be located, retrieved, presented, and interpreted. (NARA)

[12] US FDA, "*CPG Section 425.400 - Computerized Drug Processing; Input/Output Checking (CPG 7132a.07),*" September 1987.

[13] NARA Bulletin 2015-04: *Metadata Guidance.*

Additional Readings

ISO 15836-1:2017, "*Information and documentation — The Dublin Core metadata element set*" — Part 1: Core elements

UK Government, "*Data Quality and Metadata,*" in the Government Data Quality Framework, https://www.gov.uk/government/publications/the-government-data-quality-framework/the-government-data-quality-framework-guidance#data-quality-and-metadata

Chapter 13

REPORTING

INTRODUCTION

A report [1] is a document that describes the results exercises, projects or investigations, together with results, conclusions and recommendations [2].

Even with the increased use of computer systems and, subsequently, e-records, in the CGMP regulated activities, it is widespread to see regulated users rely on printouts as a hardcopy to be attached to the batch record and/or relay on printouts to perform regulated activities.

Regulatory expectation

"All data defined as critical data and associated metadata should be printable."

Aide Memoire (Ref. #: 07121202) of the German ZLG (Central Authority of the Laender for Health Protection).

Due to incorrect inputs, programming, improper mapping, configuration, computer malfunctions, or other reasons, computer printouts often contain errors. If the mistakes are unnoticed, these printouts can result in a severe production error and the distribution of an adulterated product.

If, based on the regulated user's business practices, these printouts are used as quality records, then the design, qualification and controls of these printouts are critical.

Based on the need of the regulated user, the reports are qualified as per regulated user procedural control. The functional format details in which the data were stored, should also be filed along with the data themselves.

In cases of internal audits (e.g., self-inspections [3] or external audits (e.g., inspections by regulatory agencies or competent authority), it must be possible to obtain printed reports of electronically stored data that were not specified nor validated during the implementation of the normally required reports.

In this case, to generate reliable printouts, a report generator can be utilized to take data from a source such as a database or a spreadsheet and use it to produce a document in a format that satisfies a particular human readership.

If satisfied with the computer system validation evidence, auditors can then study the computer system when it is being used and call for printouts of reports from the system and archives as relevant.

If a report generator creates the printout, then a verification of the printout must be performed before providing the printout to the auditor.

In any case, the application printout functionality must provide the capability to print audit trails [4]. In addition, EU Annex 11 [5] recommends that the printout be clear. "Clear printed" means printouts that apart from the values themselves, the units and the respective context can also be seen in the printout [6]. Units and the individual context are also known as metadata [7]

An audit trail is a form of metadata (Chapter 12) containing information associated with actions that relate to the modification or deletion of regulatory e-records [8].

In case the application printout functionality is not capable to support printing audit trails [9], it may be acceptable to describe in a procedure that additionally a printout of the related audit trail report must be generated and linked manually (e.g., paper-based revision history audit trail log) to the record [10].

Printouts must be verified before hardware and/or software is exchanged. As part of the validation/qualification of the software/ hardware, regression testing can be used to check that the data concerned can also be printed in the new configuration.

Should a change in the hardware and/or software may not allow stored data to be printed in the new configuration, then one of the following procedures should be applied [11]:

The data in the concerned format should be converted into a form that can be printed in the new configuration.

The components of the old hardware and/or software configuration required for printing should be retained. In this case, it should be guaranteed that a suitable alternative system is available in case the retained system fails.

The data is transferred to another medium.

To review, it should be possible to create an accurate copy [12] of electronic data, including relevant metadata, for review, backup and archival [8].

E-Records Reporting Requirements

The following reporting-related requirements provide meaning to e-record content. It ensures e-record integrity, usability, and audibility.

Requirement 48 - *The regulated company must have the ability to generate reports demonstrating adequate controls and compliance.*

A report records the comportment of specific exercises, projects or investigations, together with results, conclusions and recommendations.

A report needs to be properly evaluated with appropriate findings. The results and discussions need to be presented clearly in a manner that can be readily understood.

To comply with the CGMPs a report must satisfy the following five elements: written, appropriate, precise, verified, and approved. The data used to put together a report must be reliable.

- *Written.* The term 'written' means recorded or documented on media from which data may be rendered in a human-readable form [2].
- *Appropriate.* A complete report must contain a comprehensive understanding of the overall scheme or objectives.
- Personnel who do not fully understand record-keeping expectations may omit necessary information in the report.
- *Clear.* The entries of a report must be made legible and indelibly.
- In addition, a clear report is one that apart from the values themselves, the units and the respective context can also be seen in the printout [6]. Units and the particular context are considered metadata.
- *Verified.* A document is verified when the accuracy of the data can be ascertained. The person performing the verification of a document cannot prove their actions.
- *Approved.* Documented approval is necessary to ensure that responsible personnel have checked each significant step and indicated whether the operation was acceptable.
- *Reliable Data.* A reliable record is one whose content can be trusted as a complete and accurate representation of the transactions, activities, or facts to which they attest and can be depended upon during subsequent transactions or activities (NARA). A reliable report uses accurate data and can verify the report.

The US FDA requirements related to reports in the CGMP for finished pharmaceuticals can be found in 21 CFR Part 211.180 to

211.196. In the EU, the requirements for reports can be found at Good Manufacturing Practices Medicinal Products for Human and Veterinary Use Chapter 4 [2].

Requirement 49 - *The records system should provide the ability to design and generate customized reports.*

Based upon user-developed report templates or user queries, the records management application should provide the capability to generate reports on the information held within the records management application repository.

Requirement 50 - *The records system should allow print reports that are legible, professional in appearance, and usable for the regulated company official business purposes.*

Refer to this chapter section, "E-records Reporting Requirements."

Requirement 51 - *The records system should provide the ability to filter and sort report data based on the values contained in any field or column.*

A report filter screens data in your warehouse to determine whether the data should be included in or excluded from the calculations of the report results. It describes how to view a filter's definition for a given report.

Sorting a report is one of the ways data displays can be manipulated without re-executing the report against the warehouse. Sorting allows specifying the order that the data in a report for a particular row or column is presented in either ascending or descending.

Requirement 52 - *The records system should provide the ability to schedule the delivery of reports, and to distribute them to a specified list of recipients.*

A scheduled report is a report that is sent out by email at specified times. It can specify what is included, who should get the report, and how often they send it. The scheduled report may contain data for the selected time frame relative to the expected report's time to execute.

The report scheduling allows setting up specific parameters to deliver information strategically. You can set up a time frame to report during, choose the frequency (e.g., daily, weekly, monthly), and what time of the day to send it on.

It can specify what is included; who should get the report; and how often they will send it.

Requirement 53 - *The records system should provide users with the ability to design and run ad hoc reports using any information for which they have been granted access.*

It must be possible to obtain printed reports of e-records that were not specified nor validated during the implementation of the customarily required reports. These reports are configured using, as an example, Structured Query Language (SQL) language. These reports can be considered ad-hoc reports.

The access to the e-records to be reported shall be aligned with the access rights and permissions that align with the user's responsibilities performing the reporting operation.

Requirement 54 - *The records system should provide the ability to save the configurations of ad hoc reports for reuse.*

In cases of internal audits (e.g., self-inspections (Eudralex Volume 4, Chapter 9)) or external audits (e.g., inspections by regulatory agencies or competent authorities), it must be possible to obtain printed reports of e-records that were not specified nor validated during the implementation of the normally required reports. These reports are configured using, as an example, SQL language. These reports can be considered ad-hoc reports.

Ad-hoc reports can be generated using a report generator. As part of the functionality of the report, a generator is to save the configuration used to create the report.

If a report generator creates the printout, then a verification of the printout must be performed before providing the printout to the auditor/inspector.

Requirement 55 - *The records system shall provide the capability to output for viewing, saving, or printing the record profile information (metadata).*

Metadata summarizes basic data information, making finding & working with instances of data easier. Metadata can be created manually to be more accurate or automatically and contain more basic information.

Metadata is another e-record that shall be printed and viewed online. The regulated company must have the ability to generate reports of metadata.

REFERENCES

[1] López, O., "*Printouts,*" in EU Annex 11 Guide to Computer Validation Compliance for the Worldwide Health Agency GMP. López, O., Eds (CRC Press, Boca Raton, FL, 1st ed, 2015), pp. 71-73.

[2] *Eudralex*. The Rules Governing Medical Products in the European Union Volume 4 Good Manufacturing Practices Medicinal Product s for Human and Veterinary Use Chapter 4: Documentation, June 2011.

[3] *EudraLex*. Volume 4 - Good Manufacturing Practice (GMP) guidelines, Part I - Basic Requirements for Medicinal Products, Chapter 9 - Self Inspection.

[4] Computerised systems. In: *The rules governing medicinal products in the European Union.* Volume 4: Good manufacturing practice (GMP) guidelines: Annex 11 p8.2 and p9, June 2011.

[5] Computerised systems. In: *The rules governing medicinal products in the European Union.* Volume 4: Good manufacturing practice (GMP) guidelines: Annex 11 p8.1, June 2011.

[6] Journal for GMP and Regulatory Affairs, "*Q&As on Annex 11*", Issue 8, April/May 2012.

[7] Metadata - Metadata is data that describe the attributes of other data and provide context and meaning. Typically, these are data that describe the structure, data elements, inter-relationships and other characteristics of data e.g., audit trails. Metadata also permit data to be attributable to an individual (or if automatically generated, to the original data source). (CEFIC)

[8] MHRA. (March 2018). *'GxP' Data Integrity Guidance and Definitions'.*

[9] Computerised systems. In: *The rules governing medicinal products in the European Union.* Volume 4: Good manufacturing practice (GMP) guidelines: Annex 11 p8.2, June 2011.

[10] European Medicines Agency (EMEA), "*Q&A: Good Manufacturing Practices (GMP),*" February 2011.

[11] APV, "*The APV Guideline "Computerized Systems*" based on Annex 11 of the EU-GMP Guideline", Version 1.0, April 1996.

[12] ECA "*Copies in the GMP Environment - True Copies,*" ECA Academy, 02 June 2021, https://www.gmp-compliance.org/gmp-news/copies-in-the-gmp-environment-true-copies?utm_source=Newsletter&utm_medium=email&utm_campaign=ECA+GMP+Newsletter+-+2021+-+KW22+-+CEU

Chapter 14

E-RECORDS VULNERABILITIES

INTRODUCTION

The article originating this chapter was published in the GMP Journal [1]. It will be used to demonstrate how to use the DI requirements contained in Chapters 7-13 in this book with the data as a service (DaaS) application.

To successfully manage the vulnerabilities of the e-records [2], the required e-records integrity [3] controls can be categorized based on each event the e-records is performing in the e-records processing environment. These events are categorized as e-records capture, creation, processing, storing, in transit, or retrieved. These events are contained in the DI definitions in NIST [4]. These events are performed during the active and inactive e-record phases depicted in Figure 3.1, E-records Lifecycle.

The DaaS functionality determines the method on how to use these DI requirements. To facilitate the association of the corresponding requirement(s) with the associated DI function in the application, Table 1, below, will be used.

In Table 1 the NIST Lifecycle Stages and the ERM Requirements are correlated. The correlation of these two e-record lifecycles is:

Table 14.1. NIST and ERM Correlation

E-records Lifecycle Stage (NIST)	NARA Universal ERM Requirements -V2.03
Data creation	Capture and Creation
Data storage; Processing (archiving, audit trails, built-in checks, e-signature, operational checks, reports, security)	Maintenance and Use; Reporting; Metadata
Data transmission	Transfer, Metadata
Data Processing	Disposal

To facilitate the assignment of the correct ERM requirements to the DaaS function, the NIST Lifecycle Stage is to be used as a referenced. The appropriate requirement applicable to the corresponding DI function in the article will be displayed in parenthesis.

The DaaS [5] will be used as the computer environment to briefly discuss the vulnerabilities of the e-records and the applicable requirement(s).

DaaS builds on the concept that its e-records product can be provided to the regulated user [6] by a cloud service provider [7] on-demand, regardless of geographic or organizational separation between provider and consumer. In a DaaS service, the repository for e-records [8] and the e-records handling [9] are provided as a cloud service. E-records handling is a broader issue addressing potential e-records vulnerabilities. This distinction is important when evaluating technologies and the shifting roles of enterprise information technology (IT) when managing e-records in the DaaS cloud environments.

DI IN DAAS ENVIRONMENT

In the CGMP, e-records may be managed [10] in the DaaS environment (**Requirement #4**). Also, the process of managing e-records must be validated and the associated cloud infrastructure needs to be qualified by the DaaS provider based on CGMP current practices. In any case, the CGMP e-records are always owned by the regulated user.

EU Annex 11 p3 [11] and EU GMP Chapter 7 [12] provide guidelines regarding the expectations by the regulatory entities related to the efficient relationship between the DaaS provider and the regulated user (**Requirements 4, 6**).

VULNERABILITIES AND ERM REQUIREMENT

Recognizing the vulnerability in a repository for e-records, as in a DaaS, the following summarizes the vulnerabilities and actions that should be utilized to maintain the highest quality e-records level.

Discovery

In the context of the e-records processing environment, discovery is the process of examining the e-records to determine where e-records (both structured and unstructured) resides (e.g., in a database and file servers that could potentially contain regulated e-records). The outcome of this process, as an example, is the e-record sources to data target mappings. The process points to those same areas associated with DI definitions such as in NIST SP 800-57P1 [4].

A data flow diagram is a superb tool to examine the data processing environment and to map the flow of information of any process or system, including inputs, outputs, storage points, and routes between each destination. Based on this information provided by a data flow diagram, the appropriate DI controls are implemented and documented.

Figure 14.1 depicts the high-level data flow diagram. This diagram can be followed with detailed information related to each referenced area in Figure 14.1.

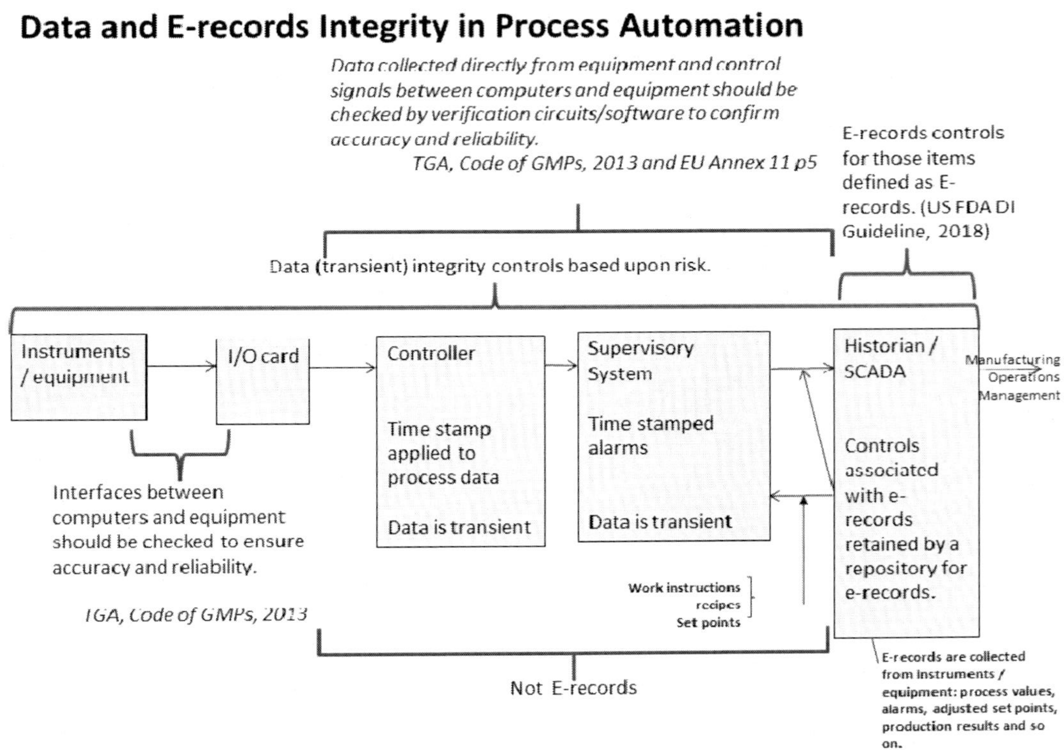

Figure 14.1. Data and E-records Integrity in Process Automation.

Data mapping and data flow diagrams are useful tools to improve data integrity. By not understanding where critical e-records [13] reside and the relevant movements, means that DI controls may not be applied in those areas where the e-records are created (Chapter 8), transmitted (Chapter 11), stored (Chapter 9), or during processing (Chapter 9). The applicable movement of the e-records is also impacted by metadata requirements (Chapter 12).

Governance

The levels defining the organizational DI philosophy can be set up in three levels. The first level is the DI Policy; the second level is the Data Governance, and the third level is the DI standard operational procedure (SOP).

The DI Policy does not need to be a broad document. It establishes the responsibilities and expectations of senior management. It should be covered the approach to quality risk management. The assessment should be based on e-records risk and e-records criticality.

The DI procedural control(s) can be explained in a procedural control.

Data governance, the subject of this section, contains the arrangements to ensure that e-records, irrespective of the format in which they are generated, are recorded, processed, retained, and used to ensure the record throughout the e-records lifecycle [14].

Data Governance (Chapter 7) must be integrated into the pharmaceutical quality system. If not integrated into the quality system, the e-records controls will not assure e-records quality. The e-records owner [15] must ensure that the governance requirements are contractually specified, and the e-records service company audited periodically to assure that the DI standards are met.

The data governance lists and summarizes all the procedural controls and, roles and responsibilities.

The governance document outlines the regulated entities' total approach to assure confidence in e-records quality [16]. The organization approach includes:

- a quality risk on DI based on e-records risk and e-records criticality. Note that e-record risks are based on vulnerabilities of the e-record. As defined before e-records criticality are e-records with high risk to product quality or patient safety. So, a quality risk on data integrity is managed by these two factors
- regulated user's roles and responsibilities
- procedural control(s) to good documentation practices
- training about e-records integrity to all electronic systems regulated users
- making accountable the senior management to support the controls associated with e-records integrity
- addressing e-records ownership and the responsibilities associated with such a role. A robust data governance approach will ensure that e-records are complete, consistent, and accurate, irrespective of the format in which e-records are generated, used or retained [17].

Data governance measures by a contract giver [18] may be significantly weakened by unreliable, falsified data or materials provided by outsourced activities. Initial and periodic audits of outsourced activities should include consideration of DI risks and appropriate control measures [19].

Cleansing

Before an integration, transformation, or migration project, the quality of the records set must be known. More frequently during the e-records lifecycle, it must be ensured as well as the e-records quality.

Cleansing is a method to detect and correct corrupt or inaccurate/inexact records from a recordset, table, or database and refers to identifying duplicate, inconsistent, incomplete, incorrect, inaccurate, or irrelevant parts of the e-records and then replacing, modifying, or deleting the dirty or coarse data. The execution of data cleansing ensures that e-records and associated metadata information are both correct and useful before analyzing the data further or starting modelling efforts.

Damaged e-records may be considered an incident and investigated to prevent it from happening again.

When an e-record is discovered to be unreadable, the e-record can be restored from a true copy of the record. If a true copy is not available, look for a trustworthy backup copy of the record and restore it from the backup set.

If the e-records set being cleansed consists of CGMP-relevant e-records, then any changes and deletions must generate an audit trail (**Requirement 43**). The reason for the modification must be documented as part of the e-record. Audit trails need to be available and convertible to a generally intelligible form and regularly reviewed [20].

In data engineering, the process of ensuring that data must go through cleansing is called data profiling. Profiling a record consists of describing the e-record content, consistency, and structure. Besides, it provides the effort needed for cleansing.

Integration

After the DaaS is deployed, the main and dangerous step is getting the extraction of the data out of a sensor or from another electronic system and loading it into the DaaS, the target system repository of e-records. Without standards and business processes the e-records across all source systems may not line up, but to resolve the situation, the data elements of the e-records can be cleansed, transformed and, as applicable, integrated.

A key element in the integration of data is the confidence in the reliability of the e-records in the source systems (**Requirement 8**).

When e-records must be shared by more than one functional activity, the standardization of e-records values is essential. Standardization of e-records value can be achieved during the e-records design. Two elements that can mitigate the integration-related vulnerability are:

- E-records profiling.
- Standardizing the format and attributes of the e-records for consistency across the regulated site/corporate. When e-records must be shared by more than one functional activity, the standardization of e-records values is essential.

Security

As a function related to security, e-records integrity service maintains information exactly as it was inputted and is auditable to affirm its reliability (**Requirements 2, 5, 17, 18, 19**).

The regulated user stores its e-records in the DaaS cloud and accesses those e-records through program interfaces. Data governance measures by a regulated user may be compromised by untrustworthy security services provided by the service provider.

A service level agreement (SLA) shall be in place between the regulated user with the service provider capturing the responsibilities of the service provider, including the e-records integrity service and the associated security.

The initial and periodic audits to the service provider and the DaaS environment must comprise DI risks and appropriate control measures.

Mastery

Mastery is the leveraging of e-records of all types to gain business insight, and then using this insight to increase revenue, decrease expenses or improve ease of doing business. It involves the use of data analytics, and big data environments to find business-relevant insights that inform better decisions for senior managers and throughout the enterprise.

Like the Capability Maturity Model in software engineering, mastery has maturity levels. Those regulated companies that have a state-of-the-art e-records management platform that leverages optimized workflows for all types of e-records are at the highest maturity level. These companies use e-records for a strategic advantage looking at hidden relationships of e-records, predictive analytics, knowledge management, and self-services.

The regulated user can start with a humble DaaS. Later, with great planning, and analytics and business intelligence DaaS may be implemented. The element of e-records quality and e-records mastery to be implemented in a humble DaaS are the same as an analytics and business intelligence DaaS, but with a complexity resulting in the incrementing the scope of the system.

SUMMARY

To set up the processes and infrastructure to manage regulated e-records, a set of technical and procedural controls must be established to maintain the reliability of each e-records after the e-record is created. It is necessary to know where the e-record resides and understand the vulnerability of the e-record to implement the correct DI-related controls.

There are six areas to evaluate the vulnerability of the e-record: discovery, governance, cleansing, integration, security, and mastery. The assessment of each of these areas provides the required DI controls to keep reliable each e-record after recording.

DISCLAIMER

Any mention of products or references to organizations is intended only to convey information; it does not imply recommendation or endorsement by Orlando López or the publisher, nor does it imply that the products mentioned are necessarily the best available for the purpose.

The opinions expressed in this article are strictly those of the author.

REFERENCES

[1] ECA (February/March 2021), "*E-records Vulnerabilities*," GMP Journal, pp 9-13.

[2] Electronic records - A collection of related data treated as a unit. (ISPE/PDA, "Good Practice and Compliance for Electronic Records and Signatures. Part 1 Good Electronic Records Management (GERM)". July 2002.)

[3] E-records integrity – A property whereby data has not been altered in an unauthorized manner since it was created, during processing, transmitted or stored. (NISP SP 800-57P1 Rev 5, "*Recommendation for Key Management, Part 1: General*," January 2016)

[4] NISP SP 800-57P1 Rev 5, "*Recommendation for Key Management, Part 1: General*," January 2016

[5] In computing, data as a service, or DaaS, is enabled by software as a service. Like all "as a service" technology, DaaS builds on the concept that its data product can be provided to the user on-demand, regardless of geographic or organizational separation between provider and consumer

[6] Regulated user - The regulated Good Practice company, that is responsible for the operation of an electronic system and the applications, files and data held thereon. The company or group is responsible for the operation of a system. The GxP customer, or user organization, contracting a supplier to provide a product. In

the context of this document, it is, therefore, not intended to apply only to individuals who use the system and is synonymous with 'Customer'. (PIC/S PI 011-3)

[7] A cloud service provider is a company that offers some components of cloud computing to other businesses or individuals.

[8] Repository for e-records - A direct access device on which the electronic records and metadata are stored.

[9] Data handling is the process of ensuring that data is created, stored, archived, or disposed of securely during the data lifecycle. (https://ori.hhs.gov/education/products/n_illinois_u/datamanagement/dmtopics.html)

[10] E-records management - The process of ensuring that data is stored, archived, or disposed of safely and securely during and after the decommissioning of the electronic system.

[11] Computerised systems. In: The rules governing medicinal products in the European Union. Volume 4: Good manufacturing practice (GMP) guidelines: Annex 11. Brussels: European Commission, June 2011. (http://ec.europa.eu/enterprise/pharmaceuticals/eudralex/vol-4/pdfs-en/anx11en.pdf).

[12] EudraLex - Volume 4 - Good Manufacturing Practice (GMP) guidelines, Part I - Basic Requirements for Medicinal Products, Chapter 7 – Outsourced Activities, January 2013.

[13] Critical e-records are e-records with high risk to product quality or patient safety. (ISPE GAMP COP Annex 11 – Interpretation, July/August 2011)

[14] E-records lifecycle – All phases in the life of the electronic record from initial generation and recording through processing (including transformation or migration), use, electronic records retention, archive/retrieval and destruction.

[15] MHRA, "*GxP Data Integrity Guidance and Definitions*," March 2018.

[16] Data quality is considered accurate, auditable, in conformance to requirement, complete, consistent, with integrity, provenance, and valid making data both correct and useful. (FIPS, Publication 11-3,

"*American National Dictionary for Information Systems*," Windrowed, July 1979.)

[17] Churchward, D., "*Good Manufacturing Practice (GMP) data integrity a new look at an old topic,*" Part 2 of 3 - MHRA Inspectorate, July 2015.

[18] Contract giver is the regulated entity owner of the data being stored by the DaaS contractor.

[19] PIC_S PI 041-1, "*Good Practice for Data Management and Integrity in Regulated GMP GDP Environments*," July 2021.

Chapter 15

INTRODUCTION TO DATA QUALITY [1]

INTRODUCTION

The "C" in CGMP stands for "current," needing companies to use technologies that are up to date to conform with the regulations.

If data integrity is the "extent to which all data are complete, consistent and accurate throughout the data lifecycle," is data integrity the knowledge up to date to fit with the regulation?

> *A plan for conducting the quality assurance process activities and tasks shall include the procedures for identification, collection, filing, maintenance, and disposition of quality records.*

The other basic concept of the US FDA is implementing a quality system to fulfil oversight and review of CGMP records. Manufacturers must develop and document control procedures to complete, secure, protect, and archive records, including data, which provide evidence of operational and quality system activities when operating under a quality system.

A quality management system (QMS) is a set of policies, processes and procedures required for planning and executing (production/ development/service) the core business area of an organization (i.e., areas that can impact the organization's ability to meet customer requirements) (ISO 9001).

The control procedures applicable to data integrity must be sufficiently comprehensive to provide evidence of operational and quality system activities.

Data is generally considered high quality if it is fit for its intended uses in operations, decision-making, and planning.

This paper discusses the significance of data quality and how it must provide accurate, valid, consistent, reliable, and complete records to support quality medicines.

DATA QUALITY

According to the Federal Information Processing Standards (FIPS), data quality is the accuracy, conformity, validity, consistency, reliability, and completeness making data both correct and valuable [2]. Refer to Figure 15.1.

The MHRA guidance [3] highlights that "This guidance primarily addresses data integrity and not data quality since the controls required for integrity do not necessarily guarantee the quality of the data generated."

The above is evident. Only four out of six dimensions defined by FIPS are contained in the data integrity guidance documents. Missing dimensions in the industry definitions are conformity and validity. Only two out of six dimensions defined by FIPS are FDA expectations. Missing dimensions in FDA expectations are conformity, validity, consistency, and completeness.

Data quality cannot exist without data reliability, and that data reliability cannot live without data integrity. Refer to Table 1.

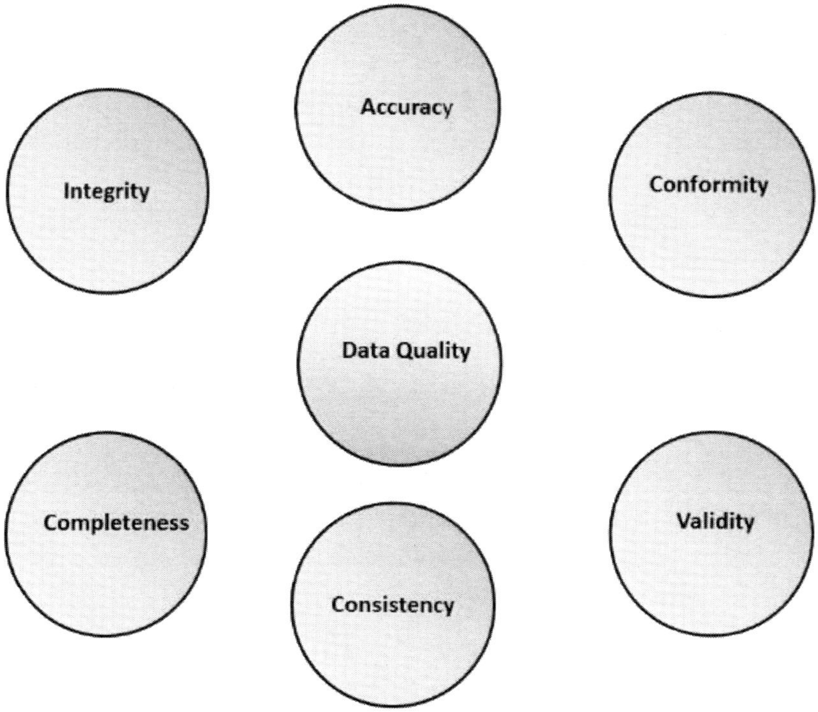

Figure 15.1. Elements of Data Quality.

Table 1. Definitions of data integrity, data reliability, and data quality

Data Integrity (NIST SP 800-57P1, ISO 17025, INFOSEC, 44 USC 3542 or ANSI/IEEE)	Data Reliability (NARA)	Data Quality (ISO 9000:2015)
The property that data has not been altered in an unauthorized manner. Data integrity covers data entry or collection, storage, transmission, and processing.	A reliable record is one whose content can be trusted as a complete and accurate representation of the transactions, activities, or facts they attest and can be depended upon in subsequent transactions or activities.	The degree to which a set of characteristics of data fulfils requirements. Examples of elements are accuracy, conformity, validity, consistency, reliability, and completeness.

The following is a brief description of each of the dimensions to data quality. It is the opinion of the author of this book that the north to the collection and management of CGMP data is the total quality of this data. ALCOA and ALCOA+ are featured in data integrity but do not provide all the elements contained in the data quality arena.

Some examples are included. These came from https://medium.com/@merwanehamadi/what-is-data-quality-55b7737f1b6e

DATA ACCURACY

It refers to whether the data values stored for an object are the correct values. Data values must be the right value and represented in a consistent and unambiguous form to be accurate. One of the dimensions in data accuracy is data reliability.

Example:

	Email address of Paul
Database	paul@gmail.com
Reality	Paul1@gmail.com

The data accuracy is designed, including the built-in checks for the correct and secure data entry and processing to minimize the risks (Annex 11-5) [4]. Data accuracy is an element of the workflows. These workflows are tested and periodically verified during the Project Stage as part of the I/O verifications.

DATA CONFORMITY

Conformity means the data follows the set of standard data definitions like data type, size and format.

Example:

Name	Unsubscribed
Paul	True
John	True
Sam	False

This workflow is designed as part of the transformation occurring before the sensor(s) signals are captured, and the data is in transient mode (Figure 3.2). These workflows are tested and periodically verified during the Project Stage as part of the I/O verifications.

DATA VALIDITY

Data validity is about the correctness and reasonableness of data.

Example:

	email
Paul	paul@g@gmail.com

As in data accuracy, this workflow is designed as part of the transformation occurring before the signals for sensor(s) are captured. The data is still in transient mode (Figure 3.2). These workflows are tested and periodically verified during the Project Stage as part of the I/O verifications.

CONSISTENCY

Consistency is the property of logical coherency among constituent parts. Consistency may also be expressed as adherence to a given set of rules.

The adherence to a given set of rules among data is designed during the Project Stage. The consistency is tested and periodically verified as part of the I/O verifications.

INTEGRITY

Data integrity is the property that data has not been altered unauthorizedly. Data integrity covers data entry or collection, storage, transmission, and processing.

The controls associated with security start early in the system's life cycle. The security requirements can be expressed as technical features (e.g., access controls), assurances (e.g., background checks for system developers), or operational practices (e.g., awareness and training). Like other system requirements, system security requirements are derived from several sources, including law, policy, applicable standards and guidelines, functional needs of the system, and cost-benefit trade-offs.

A record risk assessment looks at the sensitivity of the information to be processed. The evaluation should consider legal implications, organization policy and the functional needs of the system. Risk assessment is used to support decision-making.

System security testing includes testing the parts of the system that have been developed or acquired and the testing of the entire system. Security management, physical facilities, personnel, procedures, commercial or in-house services (such as networking services), and contingency planning are examples of areas that affect the entire system's security but may be specified outside of the development or acquisition cycle. Since only items within the development or acquisition cycle will have been tested during system acceptance testing, separate tests or reviews may need to be performed for these additional security elements.

Many security activities occur during the operational phase of a system's life. In general, these fall into three areas: security operations and administration, operational assurance, and periodic re-analysis of the security.

Access to data is controlled through data services, which tends to improve data quality, as there is a single point for updates. Only regression testing is needed once those services are tested, if they remain unchanged for the next deployment.

COMPLETENESS

The property that all necessary parts of the entity in question are included. The completeness of a product is often used to express the fact that the product has met all requirements.

DATA QUALITY DESIGN

The e-records lifecycle must incorporate two stages defining the planning, requirements and designing of the e-records model and the functionality to manage the e-records model. Refer to Chapter 3 in this book.

During the Project Stage, it should be designed to detect and prevent data defects before they corrupt databases or end-user applications.

These controls to be instituted as part of the design may include:

- Data design review.
- Accuracy checks for data entered manually. (EU Annex 11-6)
- Built-in checks for the correct and secure entry and processing data. (EU Annex 11-5)
- Until the transient data is recorded to durable media, the controls to the temporary data must ensure that the transient data may be subject to transformation but not manipulation [5].
- During the Operational Stage, implement controls the methods in which error/defect data are collected and stored for future or real-time evaluation.

- During the Operational Stage, ensuring that data will have data cleansing periodically to ensure data quality.

QUALITY CONTROL TO DATA

The e-records in storage need to be verified periodically for accessibility, readability and integrity. This process should identify incomplete, incorrect, inaccurate or irrelevant parts of the data and then replace, modify, or delete dirty or coarse data [5].

The process to correct damaged e-records provides a mechanism for creating an accurate reproduction of an original e-record that is discovered to be stained, marred, or otherwise damaged.

Data cleansing or scrubbing is the process used to ensure data quality. The error should be investigated to prevent it from happening again to correct any error.

When an e-record is discovered to be unreadable, the record can be restored from a true copy of the record. If a valid copy is not available, look for a trustworthy backup copy of the record and restore it from the backup set.

If the data set being cleansed consists of CGMP-relevant e-records, then any changes and deletions must generate an audit trail. The reason for the modification must be documented as part of the e-record. Audit trails need to be available and convertible to a generally intelligible form and regularly reviewed [6].

One method to detect integrity issues with files containing data is by using file integrity checking [7].

File integrity checkers provide a way to identify that system files have been changed, compute and store a checksum for every guarded file, and establish a file checksum database. Stored checksums are later recomputed to compare their current value with the stored value, identifying file modifications. A file integrity checker capability is usually included with any commercial host-based intrusion detection system and is also available as a standalone utility.

Although an integrity checker does not require a high degree of human interaction, it must use it carefully to ensure its effectiveness. File integrity checking is most effective when system files are compared with a reference database created using a system known to be secure—this helps ensure that the reference database was not built with compromised files. The reference database should be stored offline to prevent attackers from compromising the system and covering their tracks by modifying the database. In addition, because patches and other updates change files, the checksum database should be kept up-to-date. For file integrity checking, strong cryptographic checksums such as Secure Hash Algorithm 1 (SHA-1) should be used to ensure the integrity of e-records stored in the checksum database.

Damaged e-records may be considered an incident and investigated.

SUMMARY

A data quality assurance and data security program ensuring operations and decision-making are supported with data meeting needs of accuracy, conformity, validity, consistency, reliability, and completeness and need-to-know requirements.

Data quality can occur in a centralized place, cleansing and enriching data and offering it to different systems, applications, or users, irrespective of where they were in the organization or on the network.

Instead of regulated companies looking to develop a DI Quality Policy, creating a Data Quality Policy is suggested.

REFERENCES

[1] López, O., "Introduction to Data Quality," *Journal of Validation Technology,* Volume 26, Issue 2, April 2020.

[2] Federal Information Processing Standard (FIPS) Publication 11-3, *American National Dictionary for Information Systems,* Windrowed July 1979.

[3] MHRA, "*GxP Data Integrity and Definitions*," March 2018.

[4] Computerised systems. In: *The rules governing medicinal products in the European Union.* Volume 4: Good manufacturing practice (GMP) guidelines: Annex 11, June 2011

[5] CEFIC, "*Practical Risk-Based Guide for Managing Data Integrity*," March 2019.

[6] EU GMP Annex 11 p9, "*Computerised Systems*," June 2011.

[7] NIST, "*Technical Guide to Information Security Testing and Assessment,*" Special Publication 800-115, September 2008.

Additional Reading

Wang, R. Y., D. M. Strong, "Beyond accuracy: What data quality means to data consumers", J. Manage. Inf. Syst., vol. 12, no. 4, pp. 5-33, 1996.

Data quality refers to the state of qualitative or quantitative pieces of information. There are many definitions of data quality, but data is generally considered high quality if it is "fit for [its] intended uses in operations, decision making and planning". Moreover, data is deemed high-quality if it correctly represents the real-world construct it refers to. Furthermore, apart from these definitions, as the number of data sources increases, the question of internal data consistency becomes significant, regardless of fitness for use for any particular external purpose. People's views on data quality can often disagree, even when discussing the same set of data used for the same purpose. When this is the case, data governance is used to form agreed-upon definitions and standards for data quality. In such cases, data cleansing, including standardization, may be required to ensure data quality.

APPENDIX I: GLOSSARY OF TERMS

For additional terms, refer to the Glossary of Computerized System and Software Development Terminology[1]; A Globally Harmonized Glossary of Terms for Communicating Computer Validation Key Practices[2], EudraLex - Volume 4 Good manufacturing practice (GMP) Guidelines – Glossary[3], and the MHRA GMP Data Integrity Definitions and Guidance for Industry (March 2015).

For the purpose of this glossary, the terms and definitions given in 9000-3 and ISO 12207 are applicable. In the event of a conflict in terms and definitions, the terms and definitions specified in this glossary and the references in the first paragraph above apply.

---

[1] FDA, "*Glossary of Computerized System and Software Development Terminology*," Division of Field Investigations, Office of Regional Operations, Office of Regulatory Affairs, Food and Drug Administration, August 1995.

[2] Herr, Robert R. and Wyrick, Michael L., "*A Globally Harmonized Glossary of Terms for Communicating Computer Validation Key Practices*," PDA Journal of Pharmaceutical Science and Technology, March/April 1999.

[3] http://ec.europa.eu/health/files/eudralex/vol-4/pdfs-en/glos4en200408_en.pdf.

Abstraction.

This is a basic principle of software engineering, and enables understanding of the application and its design, and the management of complexity.

Acceptance Criteria.

The criteria that a system or component must satisfy to be accepted by a user, customer, or other authorized entity. (IEEE)

Acceptance Test.

Testing conducted to determine whether a system satisfies its acceptance criteria and to enable the customer to determine whether to accept the system. (IEEE)

Access.

The ability or opportunity to gain knowledge of stored information. (DoD 5015.2-STD)

Accuracy.

It refers to whether the data values stored for an object are the correct values. To be correct, a data values must be the right value and must be represented in a consistent and unambiguous form.

Accurate Data.

Correctly data, true, valid and reliable that reflect the recorded events/activities.

Acquirer.

An organization that acquires or procures a system, software product or software service from a supplier. (ISO 12207:1995[4])

Application.

Software installed on a defined platform/hardware providing specific functionality. (EMA Annex 11)

Application Developer.

See Software Developer.

Approver(s).

In the context of configuration management, the approver is the person(s) responsible for evaluating the recommendations of the

[4] Note: The 1995 revision is not the most recent version.

reviewers of deliverable documentation, and for rendering a decision on whether to proceed with a proposed change and initiating the implementation of a change request.

Archive.

Long term, permanent retention of completed data and relevant metadata in its final form for the purposes of reconstruction of the process or activity.

Assessment.

Investigation of processes, systems, or platforms by a subject matter expert or by IT Quality and Compliance. An assessment does not need to be independent in contrast to audit.

Audit.

An independent examination of a software product, software process, or set of software processes to assess compliance with specifications, standards, contractual agreements, or other criteria. IEEE

Auditor.

In the context of configuration management, the auditor is the person responsible for reviewing the steps taken during a development or change management process to ensure that the appropriate procedures have been followed.

Audit Trail.

An electronic means of auditing the interactions with records within an electronic system so that any access to the system can be documented as it occurs for identifying unauthorized actions in relation to the records, e.g., modification, deletion, or addition. (DOD 5015.2-STD) [2] GMP audit trails are metadata that are a record of GMP critical information (for example the change or deletion of GMP relevant data). (MHRA)

Authentication.

Verifying the identity of a user, process, or device, often as a prerequisite to allowing access to resources in an information system. (NIST Special Publication 800-18)

Authenticity.

The property of being genuine and being able to be verified and trusted; confidence in the validity of a transmission, a message, or message originator. See authentication. (NIST Special Publication 800-18)

Automated Systems.

Include a broad range of systems including, but not limited to, automated manufacturing equipment, automated laboratory equipment, process control, manufacturing execution, clinical trials data management, and document management systems. The automated system consists of the hardware, software, and network components, together with the controlled functions and associated documentation. Automated systems are sometimes referred to as computerized systems. (PICS CSV PI 011-3[5])

Availability.

Ensuring timely and reliable access to and use of information. (44 U.S.C., SEC. 3542)

Backup.

A copy of current (editable) data, metadata and system configuration settings (variable settings which relate to an analytical run) maintained for the purpose of disaster recovery. (MHRA)

Baseline.

An agreed description of the attributes of a product, at a point in time, which serves as a basis for defining change. A "change" is a movement from this baseline state to a next state.

Bespoke Computerized System.

A computerized system individually designed to suit a specific business process. (EMA Annex 11)

Best Practices.

Practices established by experience and common sense.

---

[5] PI 011-3. "Good Practices for Computerised Systems in Regulated "GXP" Environments", Pharmaceutical Inspection Co-operation Scheme (PIC/S), September 2007.

Biometrics.

Are methods of identifying a people identify based on physical measurements of an individual's physical characteristics or repeatable actions. Some examples of biometrics include identifying a user based on a physical signature, fingerprints, and so on.

Business Continuity Plan.

A plan describing how business processes will continue, respond or recover in the event of a disruption. The plan will include preparedness to meet and address emergencies and threats based on the business' prioritization of those business processes.

Business Process.

A set of structured activities or tasks that produce a specific service for a particular customer or customers. It is often visualized as a flowchart of a sequence of activities with decision points. (CEFIC)

Calibration.

Set of operations that establish, under specified conditions, the relationship between values of quantities indicated by a measuring instrument or measuring system, or values represented by a material measure or a reference material, and the corresponding values realized by standards. (PICS CSV PI 011-3)

Centrally Managed-Security System.

Computer system authentication with a centralized domain. These systems use the regulated entity network user security configuration.

Capture.

The process of placing an object under records management control for disposition and access purposes. Objects are not necessarily moved from the system they reside in when they are captured. Records can be imported from other sources, manually entered the system, or linked to other systems. (36 CFR 1236.20)

Certificate.

Certificates are used to verify the identity of an individual, organization, Web server, or hardware device. They are also used to ensure non-repudiation in business transactions, as well as enable confidentiality using public-key encryption.

Certification Authority.

As part of a public key infrastructure (PKI), an authority in a network that issues and manages from a Certificate Server security credentials and public key for message encryption and decryption. (NARA)

Certified Copy.

(1) A copy of original information that has been verified, as indicated by a dated signature, as an exact copy having all of the same attributes and information as the original. (Source: FDA, Electronic Source Data in Clinical Investigations, September 2013) (2) A copy of original information that has been verified as an exact (accurate and complete) copy having all of the same attributes and information as the original. The copy may be verified by dated signature or by a validated electronic process. (Source: CDISC (Clinical Data Interchange Standards Consortium) Clinical Research Glossary Version 8.0, December 2009)

Change.

Any variation or alteration in form, state or quality. It includes additions, deletions, or modifications impacting the hardware or software components used that affect operational integrity, service level agreements, or the validated status of applications on the system.

Change Control.

A formal system by which qualified representatives of appropriate disciplines review proposed or actual changes that might affect the validated status of facilities, systems, equipment or processes. The intent is to determine the need for action that would ensure and document that the system is maintained in a validated state. (EMA Annex 15, Qualification and Validation)

Cipher.

Series of transformations that converts plaintext to cipher text using the Cipher key.

Cipher Key.

Secret cryptography key that is used by the Key Expansion routine to generate a set of round keys.

Cipher Text.

Data output from the Cipher or input to the Inverse Cipher.

Clear Printed.

Printouts that apart from the values themselves, the units and the respective context can also be seen in the printout. (Journal for GMP and Regulatory Affairs, "Q&As on Annex 11", Issue 8, April/May 2012)

Cloud Computing.

It is the practice of using a network of remote servers hosted on the Internet to store, manage, and process data, rather than a local server or a personal computer.

Cloud Services.

Refers to technology that allows users to access and use shared data and computing services via the Internet or a Virtual Private Network (VPN). It gives users access to resources without having to build infrastructure to support these resources within their own environment or network. E-records can reside in a cloud environment hosted by a 3rd service provider (e.g., DaaS). (NARA)

Code Audit.

An independent review of source code by a person, team, or tool to verify compliance with software design documentation and programming standards. Correctness and efficiency may also be evaluated. (IEEE)

Code of Federal Regulations.

The codification of the general and permanent rules published in the Federal Register by the executive departments and agencies of the Federal Government.

Code Inspection.

A manual [formal] testing [error detection] technique where the programmer reads source code, statement by statement, to a group who ask questions analyzing the program logic, analyzing the code with respect to a checklist of historically common programming errors, and analyzing its compliance with coding standards. This technique can also be applied to other software and configuration items. (Myers/NBS)

Code Review.

A meeting at which software code is presented to project personnel, managers, users, customers, or other interested parties for comment or approval. (IEEE)

Code Walkthrough.

A manual testing [error detection] technique where program [source code] logic [structure] is traced manually [mentally] by a group with a small set of test cases, while the state of program variables is manually monitored, to analyze the programmer's logic and assumptions. (FDA Glossary of Computerized System and Software Development Technology (8/95), FDA)

Commercial of the Shelf Software.

Software commercially available, whose fitness for use is demonstrated by a broad spectrum of users. (EMA Annex 11)

Commissioning.

Refer to Site Acceptance Testing. (SAT)

Competent.

Having the necessary experience and/or training to adequately perform the job.

Completeness.

The property that all necessary parts of the entity in question are included. Completeness of a product is often used to express the fact that all requirements have been met by the product.

Complexity.

In the context of this book, complexity means the degree to which a system or component has a design or implementation that is difficult to understand and verify.

Compliance.

Compliance covers the adherence to application-related standards or conventions or regulations in laws and similar prescriptions. Fulfillment of regulatory requirements.

Compliant System.

A system that meets applicable guidelines and predicate rule requirements.

Computer.

(1) A functional unit that can perform substantial computations, including numerous arithmetic operations and logical operations without human intervention. (2) Hardware components and associated software design to perform specific functions.

Computer System.

(1) A system including the input of data, electronic processing and the output of information to be used either for reporting or automatic control. (PICS CSV PI 011-3) (2) A functional unit, consisting of one or more computers and associated peripheral input and output devices, and associated software, that uses common storage for all or part of a program and also for all or part of the data necessary for the execution of the program; executes user-written or user-designated programs; performs user-designated data manipulation, including arithmetic operations and logic operations; and that can execute programs that modify themselves during their execution. A computer system may be a stand-alone unit or may consist of several interconnected units. (ANSI)

Computer Systems Validation.

(1) The formal assessment and reporting of quality and performance measures for all the life-cycle stages of software and system development, its implementation, qualification and acceptance, operation, modification, re-qualification, maintenance and retirement. This should enable both the regulated user, and competent authority to have a high level of confidence in the integrity of both the processes executed within the controlling computer system(s) and in those processes controlled by and/or linked to the computer system(s), within the prescribed operating environment(s). (PICS

CSV PI 011-3[6]) (2) Documented evidence which provide a high degree of assurance that a computerized system analyses, controls, and records data correctly and that data processing complies with predetermined specifications. (WHO)

Computerized Process.

A process where some or all the actions are controlled by a computer.

Computerized System.

(1) A system controlled partially or totally by a computer. (2) See Automated Systems.

Computer Validation.

(1) Refer to Computer Systems Validation[7]. (2) A process of establishing and documenting that the specified requirements of a computerized system can be consistently fulfilled from design until decommissioning of the system or transition to a new system. (ICH E6(R2), section 1.65)

Concurrent Validation.

In some cases, a drug product or medical device may be manufactured individually or on a one-time basis. The concept of prospective or retrospective validation as it relates to those situations may have limited applicability. The data obtained during the manufacturing and assembly process may be used in conjunction with product testing to demonstrate that the instant run yielded a finished product meeting all its specifications and quality characteristics. (FDA)

Confidentiality.

Preserving authorized restrictions on information access and disclosure, including means for protecting personal privacy and proprietary information. (44 U.S.C., SEC. 3542)

---

[6] PI 011-3. "*Good Practices for Computerised Systems in Regulated "GXP" Environments*", Pharmaceutical Inspection Co-operation Scheme (PIC/S), September 2007.

[7] PI 011-3. "*Good Practices for Computerised Systems in Regulated "GXP" Environments*", Pharmaceutical Inspection Co-operation Scheme (PIC/S), September 2007.

Configurable Software.

Application software, sometimes general purpose, written for a variety of industries or users in a manner that permits users to modify the program to meet their individual needs. (FDA)

Configuration Item.

Entity within a configuration that satisfies an end use function and that can be uniquely identified at a giving reference point. (ISO 9000-3)

Contemporaneous E-records.

Are e-records recorded at the time they are generated.

Control System.

Included in this classification are Supervisory Control and Data Acquisition Systems (SCADA), Distributed Control Systems (DCS), Statistical Process Control systems (SPC), Programmable Logic Controllers (PLCs), intelligent electronic devices, and computer systems that control manufacturing equipment or receive data directly from manufacturing equipment PLCs.

Consistency.

The property of logical coherency among constituent parts. Consistency may also be expressed as adherence to a given set of rules.

Correctness.

The extent to which software is free from design and coding defects, i.e., fault free. It is also the extent to which software meets its specified requirements and user objectives.

Criticality.

In the context of this book, criticality means the regulatory impact to a system or component. See Critical System.

Critical.

Describes a process step, process condition, test requirement, or other relevant parameter or item that must be controlled within predetermined criteria to ensure that the product/process meets its specification.

Critical Electronic Records.

In this book critical e-records is interpreted as meaning e-records with high risk to product quality or patient safety. (ISPE GAMP COP Annex 11 – Interpretation, July/August 2011).

Critical Data.

In this book critical data is interpreted as meaning data with high risk to product quality or patient safety. (ISPE GAMP COP Annex 11 – Interpretation, July/August 2011).

Critical Deficiency.

A deficiency in a practice or process that has produced, or may result in, a significant risk of producing a product that is harmful to the user. Also occurs when it is observed that the manufacturer has engaged in fraud, misrepresentation or falsification of products or data. (TGA, Code of GMPs, 2013)

Critical Process Parameter.

A parameter which if not controlled will contribute to the variability of the end product. (Health Canada GUI-0029)

Critical Requirement.

A requirement that, if not met, has an adverse impact on any of the following: patient safety, product quality, requirements satisfying health authority regulation, cGxP data integrity or security.

Critical Step.

It is a parameter that must be within an appropriate limit, range, or distribution to ensure the safety of the subject or quality of the product of data. (MHRA)

Critical Systems.

Systems that directly or indirectly influence patient safety, product quality and data integrity.

Cryptography or cryptology.

It is the practice and study of techniques for secure communication in the presence of third parties called adversaries. (http://searchsoftwarequality.techtarget.com/definition/cryptography)

Custom Built Software.

Also known as a Bespoke System, Custom-Built Software is software produced for a customer, specifically to order, to meet a defined set of user requirements. (GAMP)

Customized Computerized System.

See Bespoke Computerized System.

Data.

Data is defined as the contents of a record. It is the basic unit of information that has a unique meaning and can be transmitted. (ISO/IEC 17025).

Information derived or obtained from raw data (e.g., a reported analytical result). (MHRA)

Database.

In electronic records, a set of data, consisting of at least one file or of a group of integrated files, usually stored in one location and made available to several users at the same time for various applications. (36 CFR 1234.2, reference (ii))

Databases refer to structured repositories of indexed information that allow information retrieval, analysis, and output. (NARA)

Database Field.

It is a place for a piece of information in a record or file.

Data Base Management System (DBMS).

A software system used to access and retrieve data stored in a database. (36 CFR 1234.2, reference (ii))

Data Collection.

The process of gathering and measuring information on variable of interest.

Data Confidentiality.

The state that exists when data is held in confidence and is protected from unauthorized disclosure. Misuse of data—by those authorized to use it for limited purposes—is also a violation of data confidentiality. (FIBS)

Data Conformity.

Conformity means the data is following the set of standard data definitions like data type, size, and format.

Data Elements.

Individual GxP data items that are part of raw data or metadata. (CEFIC)

Data Flow.

Diagram that maps the flow of information of any process or system (inputs, outputs, storage points and routes between each destination. (CEFIC)

Data Governance.

The sum of arrangements to ensure that data, irrespective the format in which it is generated, are recorded, processed, retained and used to ensure a complete, consistent and accurate record throughout the data lifecycle.

Data Handling.

The process of ensuring that data is stored, archived or disposed in a safe and secure manner during the data lifecycle.

Data Integrity.

The property that data has not been altered in an unauthorized manner since it was created, while in transit, during processing or stored. (NIST SP 800-57P1). The extent to which all data are complete, consistent and accurate throughout the data lifecycle. (IEEE and MHRA)

Data Lifecycle.

All phases in the life of the data from generation and recording through processing (including analysis, transformation or migration), use, data retention, archive/retrieval and destruction. (MHRA)

Data Mart.

A data mart is a structure/access pattern specific to data warehouse environments, used to retrieve client-facing data.

Data Migration.

Data migration is the process of transferring data between storage types, formats, or computer systems. It is a key consideration for any system implementation, upgrade, or consolidation. (Wikipedia)

Data Process Mapping.

Generation of a visual representation of the creation and movement of data through the business process including documentation of the systems used.

Data Ownership.

It refers to the possession of and responsibilities for information.

Data Quality.

Data quality is considered the accurate, auditable, in conformance to requirement, complete, consistent, with integrity, provenance, and valid making data both correct and useful. (FIPS, Publication 11-3, "American National Dictionary for Information Systems," Windrowed, July 1979.)

Data Selection.

The process of determining the appropriate data type and source, as well as suitable instruments to collect data.

Data Source.

Origin where data is collected.

Data Standards.

A set of rules about how a particular type of data should be structured, defined, formatted, or exchanged between computer systems. Data standards make submissions predictable, consistent, and have a form that an information technology system or a scientific tool can use.

Data Steward.

The person or group that manages the development, approval, and use of data within a specified functional area, ensuring that it can be used to satisfy data requirements throughout the organization. (DoD 8320.1-M-1, "Data Standardization Procedures," April 1998)

Data Transformation.

Includes data extraction, cleansing, and integration (e.g., into a Common 201 Data Model (CDM)).

Data Warehousing.

An architected, periodic and coordinated process of copying from numerous sources into an optimized environment capable of analytical and informational processing.

Data Validity.

Data validity is about the correctness and reasonableness of data.

Decommissioning.

A planned, systematic process to disassemble and retire from service a facility system and equipment without altering the integrity (validation state) of any other facility, system or equipment previously connected to the facility, system or equipment being decommissioned. The decommissioning is done via inspection, testing and documentation.

Decryption.

The transformation of unintelligible data ("ciphertext") into original data ("clear text").

Delete.

The process of permanently removing, erasing, or obliterating recorded information from a medium, especially an electronic medium.

Deliverable.

A tangible or intangible object produced as a result of project execution, as part of an obligation. In Validation Projects, Deliverables are usually documents.

Derived Data.

Data that was originally supplied in one form but was converted to another form using some automated process.

Design Qualification.

The documented verification that the proposed design of the facilities, systems and equipment is suitable for the intended purpose.

Also known as Design Verification. (EMA Annex 15, Validation and Qualification.)

Design Specification.

A specification that documents how a system is to be built. (NIST)

Developer.

An organization that performs development activities (including requirements analysis, design, testing through acceptance) during the software lifecycle process.

Development.

Software lifecycle process that contains the activities of requirements analysis, design, coding, integration, testing, installation, and support for acceptance of software products. (ISO 9000-3)

Deviation.

When a system does not act as expected.

Digital.

Pertaining to data [signals] in the form of discrete [separate/pulse form] integral values.

Digital Certificate.

A digital certificate (a.k.a also known as a public key certificate or identity certificate) is a credential issued by a trusted authority. An entity can present a digital certificate to prove its identity or its right to access information. It links a public-key value to a set of information which identifies the entity associated with the use of the corresponding private key. Certificates are authenticated, issued, and managed by a trusted third party called a CA. See also Public-key Certificates.

Digital Signature Standard (DSS).

A National Institute of Standards and Technology (NIST) standard for digital signatures, used to authenticate both a message and the signer. DSS has a security level comparable to RSA (Rivest-Shamir-Adleman) cryptography, having 1,024-bit keys.

Disaster Recovery.

The activities required to restore one or more computer systems to their valid state in response to a major hardware or software failure or destruction of facilities.

Disaster Recovery Plan.

The written and approved plan associated with a Disaster Recovery.

Discrepancy.

Any problem or entry into the Problem Reporting System. Includes all bugs and may include design issues.

Destruction.

In records management, the major type of disposal action. Methods of destroying records include selling or salvaging the record medium and burning, pulping, shredding, macerating, or discarding with other waste materials.

Disposition.

Disposition means those action taken regarding after they are no longer in office space to conduct current business. (41 CFR 201-4 and RM Handbook, references (kk) and (w))

Documentation.

1) Manuals, written procedures or policies, records, or reports that provide information concerning the uses, maintenance, or validation of a process or system involving either hardware or software. This material may be presented from electronic media. Documents include but are not limited to Standard Operating Procedures (SOPs), Technical Operating Procedures (TOPs), manuals, logs, system development documents, test plans, scripts and results, plans, protocols, and reports. Refer to Documentation and Documentation, level of in the Glossary of Computerized System and Software Development Terminology, August 1995.
2) Any written or pictorial information describing, defining, specifying, reporting or certifying activities, requirements, procedures, or results. (ANSI N45.2.10-1973)

Efficacy.

The measurement of a medicine's desired effect under ideal conditions, such as in a clinical trial.

Electronic Archive.

The designated electronic storage device in which electronic records are retained for their long-term preservation. (SAG, "A Guide to Archiving of Electronic Records," February 2014)

Electronic Record.

Information recorded in electronic form that requires a computer system to access or process. (SAG, "A Guide to Archiving of Electronic Records", February 2014)

In this book, based on the MHRA definitions, raw data and data are considered e-records. When refer to both, electronic raw data and data, it will be used the term e-records.

Electronic Record Lifecycle.

All phases in the life of the electronic record from initial generation and recording through processing (including transformation or migration), use, electronic records retention, archive/retrieval and destruction.

Electronic Records Management.

Electronic records management (ERM) is the management of electronic files and documents as records.

Electronic Source Data.

Data initially recorded in electronic format. (Source: FDA, Electronic Source Data in Clinical Investigations, September 2013)

Electronic Storage Device.

Hard drives and any form of fixed or portable storage media (e.g., network drives, CD's/DVD's, USB jump/flash drives, and other peripherals).

End User.

Personnel who use the validated computer system.

Emergency Change.

A change to a validated system that is determined to be necessary to eliminate an error condition that prevents the use of the system and interrupts the business function.

Emulation.

Refers to the process of mimicking, in software, a piece of hardware or software so that other processes think that the original equipment/function is still available in its original form. Emulation is essentially a way of preserving the functionality of and access to digital information which might otherwise be lost due to technological obsolescence.

Encryption.

(1) The process of converting information into a code or cipher so that people will be unable to read it. A secret key, or password, is required to decrypt (decode) the information. (2) Transformation of confidential plaintext into ciphertext to protect it. An encryption algorithm combines plaintext with other values called keys, or ciphers, so the data becomes unintelligible. (45 CFR 142.304)

Entity.

A software or hardware product which can be individually qualified or validated.

Establish.

Establish is defined in this book as meaning to define, document, and implement.

Evaluation.

A systematic determination of the extent to which an entity meets its specified criteria.

Exchange Format.

A data format for converting from one file or database structure to another. For example, XML is commonly used as a data exchange format.

Expected Result.

What a system should do when a particular action is performed.

Factory Acceptance Test.

An Acceptance Test in the Supplier's factory, usually involving the Customer. (IEEE)

Failure Analysis.

It is the process of collecting and analyzing data to determine the cause of a failure. One of the software-based fault location techniques is the Automatic Test Pattern Generation.

FDA Guidance Documents.

FDA guidance documents represent the FDA current thinking on a subject. These documents do not create or confer any rights for or on any person and do not operate to bind FDA or the public. An alternative approach may be used if such approach satisfies the requirements of the applicable statutes, regulations, or both.

Federal Register.

A daily issuance of the US government which provides a uniform system for making available to the public regulations and legal notices issued by Federal agencies.

Field Devices.

Hardware devices that are typically located in the field at or near the process, and which are needed to bring information to the computer or to implement a computer-driven control action. Devices include sensors, analytical instruments, transducers, and valves.

File.

An arrangement of records. The term is used to denote papers, photographs, photographic copies, maps, machine-readable information, or other recorded information regardless of physical form or characteristics, accumulated or maintained in filing equipment, boxes, or machine-readable media, or on shelves, and occupying office or storage space. (Noun) (41 CFR 201-4 and 36 CFR 1220.14, references (kk)) and (11))

Final Rule.

The regulation finalized for implementation, published in the FR (preamble and codified), and codified in the CFR.

Format.

For electronic records, the format refers to the computer file format described by a formal or vender standard or specification. For non-electronic records, the format refers to its physical form: e.g., paper, microfilm, video, and so on.

Function.

A set of specified, ordered actions that are part of a process.

Functional Requirements.

This specification describes how the system must technically operates to meet the requirements document.

Functional Testing.

Application of test data derived from the specified functional requirements without regard to the final program structure.

GMP.

Good Manufacturing Practice means the part of quality assurance which ensures that products are consistently produced and controlled in accordance with the quality standards appropriate to their intended use. (Commission Directive 2003/94/EC)

Current Good Manufacturing Practice (CGMP) refers to requirements in the Federal Food, Drug, and Cosmetic Act (FD&C Act), section 501(a)(2)(B), for all drugs and active pharmaceutical ingredients (APIs). For finished human and animal drugs, the term includes applicable requirements under 21 CFR parts 210 and 211. For biologics, the term includes additional applicable requirements under 21 CFR parts 600-680. (US FDA)

GMP Controls.

Set of controls that provide assurance of consistently continued process performance and product quality.

GMP Regulated Activities.

The manufacturing related activities **established** in the basic legislation compiled in Volume 1 and Volume 5 of the publication "The rules governing medicinal products in the European Union, US FDA 21 CFR Part 211, "Current Good Manufacturing Practice in Manufacturing, Processing, Packing or Holding of Drugs; General and Current Good Manufacturing Practice For Finished Pharmaceuticals" or any predicate rule applicable to medicinal products for the referenced country.

Good Documentation Practices.

In the context of these guidelines, good documentation practices are those measures that collectively and individually ensure documentation, whether paper or electronic, is secure, attributable, legible, traceable, permanent, contemporaneously recorded, original and accurate. (WHO)

GxP Application.

Software entities which have a specific user defined business purpose that must meet the requirements of the corresponding GxP regulation.

Guidelines.

A document providing guidance on the scientific or regulatory aspects of the development of medicines and applications for marketing authorization. Although guidelines are not legally binding, applicants need to provide justification for any deviations. (EMA)

Guidelines are departmental policy and recommended standards or statements that derive from Legislation. They do not have the force of law or regulation.

GxP Computerized Systems.

A computer system that performs a regulated operation which is required to be formally controlled under a GXP international life science requirement.

GxP Regulation.

A global abbreviation intended to cover GMP, GCP, GLP, and other regulated applications in context.

The underlying international life science requirements such as those set forth in the US FD&C Act, US PHS Act, FDA regulations, EU Directives, Japanese MHL.W regulations, Australia TGA, or other applicable national legislation or regulations under which a company operates. (GAMP Good Practice Guide, IT Infrastructure Control and Compliance, ISPE 2005)

Human Readable.

An electronic record, data or signature that can be displayed in a viewable form, e.g., on paper or computer screen and has meaning (words in a written language).

Hybrid Systems.

Hybrid computer systems include combinations of paper records (or other nonelectronic media) and electronic records, paper records and electronic signatures, or handwritten signatures executed to electronic records.

Ingestion.

The process that accepts electronic records for archiving. (SAG, "A Guide to Archiving of Electronic Records," February 2014)

Information.

Facts provided or learned about something or someone.

Information security.

It is a set of strategies for managing the processes, tools and policies necessary to prevent, detect, document and counter threats to digital and non-digital information. Infosec responsibilities include establishing a set of business processes that will protect information assets regardless of how the information is formatted or whether it is in transit, is being processed or is at rest in storage.

Information Technology.

Any equipment or interconnected system or subsystem of equipment that is used in the automatic acquisition, storage, manipulation, management, movement, control, display, switching, interchange, transmission, or reception of data or information by the executive agency. For purposes of the preceding sentence, equipment is used by an executive agency if the equipment is used by the executive agency directly or is used by a contractor under a contract with the executive agency which: (i) requires the use of such equipment; or (ii) requires the use, to a significant extent, of such equipment in the performance of a service or the furnishing of a product. The term information technology includes computers, ancillary equipment, software, firmware and similar procedures, services (including support services), and related resources. (40 U.S.C., SEC. 1401)

Infrastructure.

The hardware and software, such as networking software and operation systems, which makes it possible for the application to function. (EMA Annex 11)

Interface.

A shared boundary. To interact or communicate with another system component. (ANSI/IEEE)

Impact of change.

The impact of change is the effect of the change on the GXP computer system. The components by which the impact of change is evaluated may include, but not be limited to, business considerations; resource requirements and availability; application of appropriate regulatory agency requirements; and criticality of the system.

Inspection.

(1) A manual testing technique in which program documents [specifications (requirements, design), source code or user's manuals] are examined in a very formal and disciplined manner to discover any errors, violations of standards or other problems. Checklists are typical vehicles used in accomplishing this process. (2) A visual examination of a software product to detect and identify software anomalies, including errors and deviations from standards and specifications. Inspections are peer examinations led by impartial facilitators who are trained in inspection techniques. Determination of remedial or investigative action for an anomaly is a mandatory element of a software inspection, although the solution should not be determined in the inspection meeting.

Installation Qualification.

Establishing confidence that process equipment and ancillary systems are capable of consistently operating within established limits and tolerances. (FDA)

Integration Testing.

Orderly progression of testing in which software elements, hardware elements, or both, are combined and tested, until all inter-module communication links have been integrated.

Integrity.

Guarding against improper information modification or destruction and includes ensuring information non-repudiation and authenticity. (44 U.S.C., Sec. 3542). (2) Protection against unauthorized changes to information. (3) Condition existing when data is unchanged from its source and has not been accidentally or maliciously modified, altered, or destroyed. (National Information System Security (INFOSEC) Glossary) (4) The degree to which a system or component prevents unauthorized access to, or modification of, computer programs or data. (ANSI/IEEE)

Intended Use.

Use of a product, process or service in accordance with the specifications, instructions and information provided by the manufacturer. (ANSI/AAMI/ISO 14971) (2) Refer to the objective intent of the persons legally responsible for the labeling of devices. The intent is determined by such persons' expressions or may be shown by the circumstances surrounding the distribution of the article. This objective intent may, for example, be shown by labeling claims, advertising matter, or oral or written statements by such persons or their representatives. It may be shown by the circumstances that the article is, with the knowledge of such persons or their representatives, offered and used for a purpose for which it is neither labeled nor advertised. The intended uses of an article may change after it has been introduced into interstate commerce by its manufacturer. If, for example, a packer, distributor, or seller intends an article for different uses than those intended by the person from whom he received the devices, US FDA Draft Guidance for Industry and Food and Drug Administration Staff - Mobile Medical Applications, July 2011.

IT Infrastructure.

The hardware and software such as networking software and operation systems, which makes it possible for the application to function. (EMA Annex 11)

Key Practices.

Processes essential for computer validation that consists of tools, workflow, and people. (PDA)

Legacy Systems.

Production computer systems that are operating on older computer hardware or are based on older software applications. In some cases, the vendor may no longer support the hardware or software. (2) These are regarded as systems that have been established and in use for some considerable time. For a variety of reasons, they may be generally characterized by lack of adequate GMP compliance related documentation and records pertaining to the development and commissioning stage of the system. Additionally, because of their age there may be no records of a formal approach to validation of the system. (PICS CSV PI 011-3[8])

Lifecycle Model.

A framework containing the processes, activities, and tasks involved in the development, operation, and maintenance of a software product, spanning the life of the system from the definition of its requirements to the termination of its use. (ISO 9000-3)

Lifecycle (record).

The life span of a record from its creation to its final disposition is considered its lifecycle. There are four stages in a record lifecycle: Creation, Maintenance, Retention Management and Disposal.

Limited Security System.

Computer system with limited security functionality, such as but not limited to: non-individual accounts, limited number of users, and security based on group-passwords.

---

[8] PI 011-3. "*Good Practices for Computerised Systems in Regulated "GXP" Environments*", Pharmaceutical Inspection Co-operation Scheme (PIC/S), September 2007.

Living Document.

A document (or collection of documents) revised as needed throughout the life of a computer system. Only the most recent version(s) is effective and supersedes prior versions.

Locally Managed-Security System.

Computer system locally authenticated (e.g., with a local domain or a stand-alone system), in which the security process. These systems use equipment specific user security configuration and do not use the regulated entity network user security configuration.

Logically Secure and Controlled Environment.

A computing environment, controlled by policies, procedures, and technology, which deters direct or remote unauthorized access which could damage computer components, production applications and/or data.

Lifecycle.

All phases in the life of the system from initial requirements until retirement including design, specification, programming, testing, installation, operation, and maintenance. (EMA Annex 11)

Lifecycle Model.

Framework containing the processes, activities, and tasks involved in the development, operation, and maintenance of a software product, spanning the life of the system from the definition of its requirements to the termination of its use. (ISO 9000-3)

Maintainer.

An organization that performs maintenance activities. (ISO 12207:19954)

Major Change.

A change to a validated system that is determined by reviewers to require the execution of extensive validation activities.

Manufacture.

All operations of purchase of materials and products, Production, Quality Control, release, storage, dispatch of medicinal products and the related controls.

Manufacturer.

An entity that engages in CGMP activities, including implementation of oversight and controls over the manufacture of drugs to ensure quality.

Manufacturing.

All operations of receipt of materials, production, packaging, repackaging, labeling, relabeling, quality control, release, storage and distribution of medicinal products and the related controls.

Manufacturing Systems.

Elements of pharmaceutical and biopharmaceutical manufacturing capability, including manufacturing systems, facility equipment, process equipment, supporting utilities, associated process monitoring and control systems, and automation systems, that have the potential to affect product quality and patient safety. (ASTM E 2500 – 07)

Mapping.

The process of creating data element linkages between two distinct data models.

May.

This word, or the adjective "OPTIONAL", mean that an item is truly optional. Statement using "may" for permissible actions.

Metadata.

Data describing stored data: that is, data describing the structure, data elements, interrelationships, and other characteristics of electronic records. (DOD 5015.2-STD) Data that describe the attributes of other data and provide context and meaning. Typically, these are data that describe the structure, data elements, interrelationships and other characteristics of data. It also permits data to be attributable to an individual. (MHRA)

Migration.

The act of moving records from one system to another.

Minor Change.

A change to a validated system that is determined by reviewers to require the execution of only targeted qualification and validation activities.

Model.

A model is an abstract representation of a given object.

Module Testing.

Refer to Testing, Unit in the Glossary of Computerized System and Software Development Terminology, August 1995.

Native file format.

It is a method used by the computer operating system or file management to arrange data.

NEMA Enclosure.

Hardware enclosures (usually cabinets) that provide different levels of mechanical and environmental protection to the devices installed within it.

Non-Conformance.

A departure from minimum requirements specified in a contract, specification, drawing, or other approved product description or service.

Non-Custom Purchased Software Package.

A generally available, marketed software product, which performs specific data collection, manipulation, output, or archiving functions. Refer to Configurable, off-the-shelf software in the Glossary of Computerized System and Software Development Terminology, August 1995.

Non-Repudiation.

Strong and substantial evidence of the identity of the signer of a message and of message integrity, enough to prevent a party from successfully denying the origin, submission or delivery of the message and the integrity of its contents.

Objective Evidence.

Qualitative or quantitative information, records or statements of fact pertaining to the quality of an item or service or to the existence of a quality system element, which is based on observation, measurement or test and which can be verified.

Operator.

An organization that operates the system. (ISO 12207:19954)

Operating Environment.

All outside influences that interface with the computer system. (GAMP)

Ongoing Evaluation.

A term used to describe the dynamic process employed after a system's initial validation that can assist in maintaining a computer system in a validated state.

Operational Testing.

Refer to Operational Qualification in the Glossary of Computerized System and Software Development Terminology, August 1995.

Operating System.

Software that controls the execution of programs and that provides services such as resource allocation, scheduling, input/output control, and data management. Usually, operating systems are predominantly software, but partial or complete hardware implementations are possible. (ISO)

Original Record.

Data as the file or format in which it was originally generated, preserving the integrity (accuracy, completeness, content and meaning) of the record, e.g., original paper record of manual observation, or electronic raw data file from a computerized system (MHRA)

Part 11 Records.

Records that are required to be maintained under predicate rule requirements and that are maintained in electronic format in place of paper format, or records that are required to be maintained under predicate rules, that are maintained in electronic format in addition to paper format, and that are relied on to perform regulated activities. Part 11 records include records submitted to FDA, under predicate rules (even if such records are not specifically identified in Agency regulations) in electronic format (assuming the records have been identified in docket number 92S-0251 as the types of submissions the Agency accepts in electronic format). (FDA guidance: Part 11 Scope and Application)

Password.

A character string used to authenticate an identity. Knowledge of the password that is associated with a user ID is considered proof of authorization to use the capabilities associated with that user ID. (CSC-STD-002-85)

Packaged Software.

Software provided and maintained by a vendor/supplier, which can provide general business functionality or system services. Refer to Configurable, off-the-shelf software in the Glossary of Computerized System and Software Development Terminology, August 1995.

Periodic Review.

A documented assessment of the documentation, procedures, records, and performance of a computer system to determine whether it is still in a validated state and what actions, if any, are necessary to restore its validated state. (PDA) The review is performed at a regular interval. The timing of intervals is left flexible.

Persisted Data/E-record.

Persisted E-records - E-records residing in the diverse data warehouses acquired from a source system(s).

Person.

By "person", it refers to an individual or an organization with legal rights and duties.

Personal Identification Number.

A PIN is an alphanumeric code or password used to authenticate the identity of an individual.

Physical Environment.

The physical environment of a computer system that comprises the physical location and the environmental parameters in which the system physically functions.

Planned Change.

An intentional change to a validated system for which an implementation and evaluation program is predetermined.

Policy.

A directive which usually specifies what is to be accomplished.

Preamble.

Analysis preceding a proposed or final rule that clarifies the intention of the rulemaking and any ambiguities regarding the rule. Responses to comments made on a proposed rule are published in the preamble preceding the final rule. Preambles are published only in the FR and do not have a binding effect.

Predicate Regulations.

Federal Food, Drug, and Cosmetic Act, the Public Health Service Act or any FDA Regulation, except for 21 CFR Part 11. Predicate regulations address the research, production, and control of FDA regulated articles.

Preservation.

Ensuring that electronic records held in the archive remain accessible through the application of appropriate preservation policies and processes. In the context of electronic archiving this means maintenance of the authenticity and integrity of e-records. (SAG, "A Guide to Archiving of Electronic Records," February 2014)

Primary Record.

The record which takes primacy in cases were collected or retained concurrently by more than one method fail to concur. (MHRA)

Principles.

A foundation of believes, truths, and so on, upon which others are based.

Procedural Controls.

(1) Written and approved procedures providing appropriate instructions for each aspect of the development, operations, maintenance, and security applicable to computer technologies. In the context of regulated operations, procedural controls should have QA/QC controls that are equivalent to the applicable predicate

regulations. (2) A directive usually specifying how certain activities are to be accomplished. PMA CSVC

Process.

A set of specified, ordered actions required to achieve a defined result.

A set of interrelated or interacting activities that transform input into outputs. (ISO 9000-3)

Process Owner.

The person responsible for the business process. (EMA Annex 11)

Process Mapping.

Activities involved in defining what a business entity does, who is responsible, to what standard a business process should be completed, and how the success of a business process can be determined. (CEFIC)

Process System.

The combination of the process equipment, support systems (such as utilities), and procedures used to execute a process.

Processable Electronic Records.

Records in native file formats that can be read, analyzed, interpreted, and manipulated by current and future hardware and software that can be read the native file structure.

Processing Environment.

The environment in which the e-records were initially created. (ISPE/PDA, "Technical Report: Good Electronic Records Management (GERM)," July 2002)

Production Environment.

The operational environment in which the system is being used for its intended purpose, i.e., not in a test or development environment.

Production Verification (PV).

Documented verification that the integrated system performs as intended in its production environment. PV is the execution of selected Performance Qualification (PQ) tests in the production environment using production data.

Project.

A project is an activity which achieves specific objectives through a set of defining tasks and effective use of resources.

Project Management.

Project management is the application of knowledge, skills, tools, and techniques to project activities to meet the project requirements. (ANSI)

Prospective Validation.

Validation conducted prior to the distribution of either a new product, or product made under a revised manufacturing process, where the revisions may affect the product's characteristics. (FDA)

Public-key Certificate.

A public key certificate (a.k.a. a digital certificate or identity certificate) is an electronic representation of an identification or passport, issued by a certification authority (CA) to a PKI user, stating identification information, validity period, the holder's public key, the identity and digital signature of the issuer, and the purpose for which it is issued. (GERM)

Qualification.

(1) Action of proving that any equipment works correctly and leads to the expected results. The word validation is sometimes widened to incorporate the concept of qualification. (PIC/S) (2) Qualification is the process of demonstrating whether a computer system and associated controlled process/operation, procedural controls, and documentation can fulfill specified requirements. (3) The process of demonstrating whether an entity can fulfill specified requirements. (ISO 8402: 1994, 2.13.1) (4) Describes verification of system functionality. (Notice to sponsors on validation and qualification of computerized systems used in clinical trials EMA/INS/GCP/ 467532/2019) (4) The action of proving that any equipment works correctly and consistently and produces the expected results. Qualification is part of, but not limited to, a validation process, i.e., installation qualification (IQ), operational qualification (OQ), and

performance qualification (PQ). (Draft API GMP Guide, September 1997 (Draft))

Qualification Protocol.

A prospective experimental plan stating how qualification will be conducted, including test parameters, product characteristics, production equipment, and decision points on what constitutes an acceptable test. When executed, a protocol is intended to produce documented evidence that a system or subsystem performs as required.

Quality and Technical Records.

Registered evidence about activities on the QMS and/or the process of performing tests (e.g., work sheets, logbooks, control graphs, documentation of equipment qualification, test requests, test reports, reports from audits, training records, records of corrective and preventive actions, and so on.). (OMLC - Management of Documents and Records (Rephrased))

Qualification Reports.

These are test reports which evaluate the conduct and results of the qualification carried out on a computer system.

Quality.

The totality of features and characteristics of a product or service that bears on its ability to satisfy given needs.

Quality Assurance.

All planned and systematic activities implemented within the quality system and demonstrated as needed to provide adequate confidence that an entity will fulfil requirements for quality.

Quality Management.

All activities of the overall management function that determine the quality policy, objectives, and responsibilities and implement them by such means as quality planning, quality control, quality assurance, and quality improvement within the quality system.

Quality System.

To establish policy and objectives and to achieve those objectives to direct and control an organization regarding quality. (ISO 9000:2015)

Raw Data.

All data on which quality decisions are based should be defined as raw data. It includes data which is used to generate other records. (Source: Volume 4, EU Good Manufacturing Practice Medicinal Poducts for Human and Veterinary Use, Chapter 4: Documentation)

Original records and documentation, retained in the format in which they were originally generated (i.e., paper or electronic), or as a "true copy". In the case of basic electronic equipment which does not store data, or the printout constitutes the raw data. Raw data must be contemporaneously and accurately recorded by permanent means. (MHRA) The raw data must be permanent, protected against unauthorized modification, written to durable storage location contemporaneously, and must reflect the actual observation.

Any laboratory worksheets, records, memoranda, notes, or exact copies thereof that are the result of original observations and activities of a nonclinical laboratory study and are necessary for the reconstruction and evaluation of the report of that study. If exact transcripts of raw data have been prepared (e.g., tapes which have been transcribed verbatim, dated, and verified accurate by signature), the exact copy or exact transcript may be substituted for the original source as raw data. Raw data may include photographs, microfilm or microfiche copies, computer printouts, magnetic media, including dictated observations, and recorded data from automated instruments. (Source: US FDA 21 CFR 58.3(k))

Record.

A collection of related data treated as a unit. (GERM)

The record provides evidence of various actions taken to demonstrate compliance with instructions, e.g., activities, events, investigations, and in the case of manufactured batches a history of each batch of product, including its distribution. Records include the raw data which is used to generate other records. For electronic records regulated users should define which data are to be used as raw data. At least, all data on which quality decisions are based should be defined as raw data. (Eudralex Vol 4 Ch 4)

A record consists of information, regardless of medium, detailing the transaction of business. Records include all books, papers, maps, photographs, machine-readable materials, and other documentary materials, regardless of physical form or characteristics, made or received by an Agency of the United States Government under Federal law or in connection with the transaction of public business and preserved or appropriate for preservation by that Agency or its legitimate successor as evidence of the organization, functions, policies, decisions, procedures, operations, or other activities of the Government or because of the value of data in the record. (44 U.S.C. 3301, reference (bb))

Record Keeping.

The field of management responsible for the efficient and systematic control of the creation, receipt, maintenance, use and disposition of records, including the processes for capturing and maintaining evidence of and information about business activities and transactions in the form of records. (ISO 15489: 2001)

Record Management.

The planning, controlling, directing, organizing, training, promoting, and other managerial activities involving the lifecycle of information, including creation, maintenance (use, storage, retrieval), and disposal, regardless of media. Record management procedures are used to achieve adequate and proper documentation of Federal policies and transactions and effective and economical management of Agency/organizational operations. (44 U.S.C. 2901)

Record Owner.

"Record Owner" means a person or organization who can determine the contents and use of the data collected, stored, processed or disseminated by that party regardless of whether the data was acquired from another owner or collected directly from the provider.

Record Reliability.

A reliable record is one whose contents can be trusted as a full and accurate representation of the transactions, activities, or facts to which they attest and can be depended upon in the course of subsequent transactions or activities. (NARA)

Record Retention Period.

Length of time the electronic record is to be retained, as mandated by the requirement of the record type, based on regulations or documented policies.

Record Retention Schedule.

A list of record types with the required storage conditions and defined retention periods. The time (retention) periods are established based upon regulatory, legal and tax compliance requirements as well as operational need and historical value.

Reengineering.

The process of examining and altering an existing system to reconstitute it in a new form. May include reverse engineering (analyzing a system and producing a representation at a higher level of abstraction, such as design from code), restructuring (transforming a system from one representation to another at the same level of abstraction), documentation (analyzing a system and producing user or support documentation), forward engineering (using software products derived from an existing system, together with new requirements, to produce a new system), retargeting (transforming a system to install it on a different target system), and translation (transforming source code from one language to another or from one version of a language to another). (DOD-STD-498)

Regulated Data.

Information used for a regulated purpose or to support a regulated process (GAMP). (2) Data used for GMP purposes as required by the Rules GMP related to operations that may affect patient safety and product quality (Russian SIDGP Data Integrity Guidance (August 2018).

Regulated Record.

It is a record required to be maintained or submitted by GxP regulations.

Regulated Electronic Records.

It is a regulated record maintained in electronic format.

Regulations.

Regulations are rules for following and enforcing the law. US FDA enforces the regulations contained in Title 21 CFR.

Reports.

Document the conduct of exercises, projects or investigations, together with results, conclusions and recommendations (Eudralex Vol 4 Ch 4). A report containing regulated data is considered a regulated record..

Reliability.

A record is reliable if its content can be trusted as a full and accurate representation of the transaction, activities, or facts to which it attests, and it can be depended upon in the course of subsequent transactions and activities. (NARA)

Repository for Electronic Records.

A direct access device on which the electronic records and metadata are stored.

Regression Testing.

Regression testing is the process of testing changes to computer programs to make sure that the older programming still works with the new changes. Regression testing is a normal part of the program development process and, in larger companies, is done by code testing specialists. Test department coders develop code test scenarios and exercises that will test new units of code after they have been written. These test cases form what becomes the test bucket. Before a new version of a software product is released, the old test cases are run against the new version to make sure that all the old capabilities still work. The reason they might not work is because changing or adding new code to a program can easily introduce errors into code that is not intended to be changed.

Regulated Operations.

Process/business operations carried out on a regulated agency product that is covered in a predicated rule.

Regulated User.

The regulated Good Practice entity, that is responsible for the operation of a computerized system and the applications, files and data held thereon. (PIC/S PI 011-3) See Also 'User' and 'Operator.'

Regulation.

Regulations are rules for following and enforcing the law. FDA enforces all the regulations contained in Title 21 CFR.

Regulatory Authorities.

Bodies having the statutory power to regulate. The expression "regulatory authorities" includes the authorities that review submitted products data and conduct inspections.

Regulatory Requirements.

Any part of a law, ordinance, decree, or other regulation which applies to the regulated article.

Release.

Version of a configuration item that is made available for a specific purpose. (ISO 9000-3)

The ability of a system or component to perform its required functions under stated conditions for a specified period. (American National Standards Institute/The Institute of Electrical and Electronics Engineers, Inc. (IEEE) Std 610.12-1990, IEEE Standard Glossary of Software Engineering Terminology)

Reliable Records.

Records that are a full and accurate representation of the transactions, activities or facts to which they attest and can be depended upon in the course of subsequent transactions or activities.

Remediate.

In the context of this book, the software, hardware and/or procedural changes employed to bring a system into compliance with the applicable GXP rule.

Remediation Plan.

A documented approach on bringing existing computer systems into compliance with the regulation/s.

Replacement.

The implementation of a new compliant system after the retirement of an existing system.

Re-qualification.

Repetition of the qualification process or a specific portion thereof.

Requirement.

A condition or capability that must be met or possessed by a system or system component to satisfy a contract, standard, specification, or other formally imposed document. The set of all requirements forms the basis for subsequent development of the system or system component. (ANSI/IEEE)

Retention Environment.

The environment used for subsequent safe keeping and preservation of the e-records. (GERM)

Retention Period.

- The length of time specified for data on a data medium to be preserved. (ISO)
- The duration for which records are retained. Retention periods are defined in a retention schedule document. This retention schedules are based on business requirements, country-specific regulatory and legal requirements.

Retirement Phase.

The period in the SLC in which plans are made and executed to decommission or remove a computer technology from operational use.

Retrospective Evaluation.

Establishing documented evidence that a system does what it purports to do based on an analysis of historical information. The process of evaluating a computer system, which is currently in operation, against standard validation practices and procedures. The evaluation determines the reliability, accuracy, and completeness of a system.

Retrospective Validation.

See Retrospective Evaluation.

Revision.

Different versions of the same document. Can also be used in reference to software, firmware and hardware boards. Implies a fully tested, fully functional and released unit/component/document.

Risk.

A measure of the extent to which an organization is threatened by a potential circumstance or event, and typically a function of the following:

- The adverse impacts that would arise if the circumstance or event occurs; and
- The likelihood of occurrence. Likelihood is influenced by the ease of exploit(s) required and the frequency with which an exploit or like-objects are being attacked at present. (K. Dempsey, P. Eavy and G. Moore, "Automation Support for Security Control Assessments Volume 1: Overview," Draft NISTIR 8011, February 2016.)

Risk Assessment.

A comprehensive evaluation of the risk and its associated impact.

Risk Management.

The tasks and plans that help avoid risk and helps minimize damage.

Review.

A process or meeting during which a software product is presented to project personnel, managers, users, customers, user representatives, or other interested parties for comment or approval. (IEEE)

SAT.

Inspection and/or dynamic testing of the systems or major system components to support the qualification of an equipment system conducted and documented at the manufacturing site.

Secure Repository.

A repository or application that, in accordance with specific country laws and regulations, permits users to securely store records and limits the ability to edit and delete documents.

Security Controls.

The management, operational, and technical controls (i.e., safeguards or countermeasures) prescribed for an information system to protect the confidentiality, integrity, and availability of the system and its information.

Self-inspection.

An audit carried out by people from within the organization to ensure compliance with GMP and regulatory requirements.

Segregation of Duties.

A process that divides roles and responsibilities so that a single individual cannot subvert a critical process.

Service Provider.

An organization supplying services to one or more internal or external customers. (ITIL Service Design, 2011 Edition)

Shall.

Used to express a provision that is binding, per regulatory requirement. Statements that use "shall" can be traced to a regulatory requirement and must be followed to comply with such requirements. (RFC 2119, RFC Key Words, March 1997).

Should.

Used to express a non-mandatory provision. Statements that use "should" are best practices, recommended activities, or options to perform activities to be considered in order to achieve quality projects results. Other methods may be used if it can be demonstrated that they are equivalent. (RFC 2119, RFC Key Words, March 1997).

SIPOC Diagram.

It is a tool used to identify all significant elements of a process. The representation of such process is a high-level process map.

Signature, Handwritten.

The scripted name or legal mark of an individual handwritten by that individual and executed or adopted with the present intention to authenticate a writing in a permanent form. (21 CFR 11.3(8))

Site.

In this book "Site" is used to indicate where local guidelines, standards, procedures and organizations underpin a global policy.

Site Acceptance Test.

An Acceptance Test at the Customer's site, usually involving the Customer. (IEEE)

Software Developer.

Person or organization that designs software and writes the programs. Software development includes the design of the user interface and the program architecture as well as programming the source code. (TechWeb Network, http://www.techweb.com/encyclopedia/)

Software Development Standards.

Written policies or procedures that describes practices a programmer or software developer should follow in creating, debugging, and verifying software.

Software Item.

Identifiable part of a software product. (ISO 9000-3)

Software Product.

Set of computer programs, procedures, and possibly associated documentation and data. (ISO 9000-3)

Source Code.

The human readable version of the list of instructions (programs) that enable a computer to perform a task.

Source Data.

All information in original records and certified copies of original records of clinical findings, observations, or other activities in a clinical trial necessary for the reconstruction and evaluation of the trial. Source data are contained in source documents (original records or certified copies). (Source: EMA/INS/GCP/454280/2010 GCP Inspectors Working Group (GCP IWG). Reflection paper on expectations for electronic source data and data transcribed to electronic data collection)

All information in original records and certified copies of original records of clinical findings, observations, or other activities (in a clinical investigation) used for the reconstruction and evaluation of the trial. Source data are contained in source documents (original records or certified copies). (Source: FDA, Electronic Source Data in Clinical Investigations, September 2013)

Specification.

A document that specifies, in a complete, precise, verifiable manner, the requirements, design, behavior, or other characteristics of a system or component, and often, the procedures for determining whether these provisions have been satisfied. (IEEE)

Stakeholder.

In this book, anyone who has a stake in the successful outcome of the project – system owner(s), business managers, regulated end-users, quality assurance, software engineers, support people, and so forth.

Static Analysis.

(1) Analysis of a program that is performed without executing the program. (NBS) (2) The process of evaluating a system or component based on its form, structure, content, documentation. (IEEE)

Standard Instrument Software.

These are driven by non-user-programmable firmware. They are configurable. (GAMP)

Standard Operation Procedures.

See Procedural Controls.

Standard Software Packages.

A complete and documented set of programs supplied to several users for a generic application or function. (ISO/IEC 2382-20:1990)

Structured Data.

Refers to data that is stored in defined fields. Categories for structured data include database formats, spreadsheets, statistical data that is the result of quantitative research and analysis, and scientific data collected by instrumentation tools during the scientific process.

Subject Matter Experts.

Individuals with specific expertise and responsibility in a particular area or field. (ASTM, E 2500 – 07 Standard Guide for Specification,

Design, and Verification of Pharmaceutical and Biopharmaceutical Manufacturing Systems and Equipment)

Supplier.

An organization that enters into a contract with the acquirer for the supply of a system, software product or software service under the terms of the contract. (ISO 12207:19954)

System.

(1) People, machines, and methods organized to accomplish a set of specific functions. (ANSI) (2) A composite, at any level of complexity, of personnel, procedures, materials, tools, equipment, facilities, and software. The elements of this composite entity are used together in the intended operational or support environment to perform a given task or achieve a specific purpose, support, or mission requirement. (DOD). (3) A group of related objects designed to perform or control a set of specified actions.

System Backup.

The storage of data and programs on a separate media and stored separately from the originating system.

System Documentation.

The collection of documents that describe the requirements, capabilities, limitations, design, operation, and maintenance of an information processing system. See: specification, test document-tation, user's guide. (ISO)

System Integrity.

The quality that a system has when it performs its intended function in an unimpaired manner, free from unauthorized manipulation. (NIST SP 800-33, Withdrawn: August 20182018)

System Lifecycle.

All phases in the life of the system from initial requirements until retirement including design, specification, programming, testing, installation, operation, and maintenance. (EMA Annex 11)

System Owner.

The person responsible for the availability, and maintenance of a computerized system and for the security of the data residing on that system. (EMA Annex 11)

System Retirement.

The removal of a system from operational usage. The system may be replaced by another system or may be removed without being replaced.

System Software.

See Operating System.

System Specification.

In this book system specification corresponds to requirements, functional and/or design specifications. Refer to Specification.

System Test.

Process of testing an integrated hardware and software system to verifythat the system meets its specified requirements.

Technological Controls.

Are program enforcing compliance rules.

Templates.

Guidelines that outline the basic information for a specific set of equipment. (JETT)

Test Report.

Document that presents test results and other information relevant to a test. (ISO/IEC Guide 2:2004)

Test Script.

A detailed set of instructions for execution of the test. This typically includes the following:

- Specific identification of the test
- Prerequisites or dependencies
- Test objective
- Test steps or actions
- Requirements or instructions for capturing data (e.g., screen prints, report printing)
- Pass/fail criteria for the entire script

- Instructions to follow if a non-conformance is encountered
- Test execution date
- Person(s) executing the test
- Review date

Person reviewing the test results.

For each step of the test script, the item tested, the input to that step, and the expected result are indicated prior to execution of the test. The actual results obtained during the steps of the test are recorded on or attached to the test script. Test scripts and results may be managed through computer-based electronic tools. Refer to Test case in the Glossary of Computerized System and Software Development Terminology, August 1995.

Test Non-Conformance.

A non-conformance occurs when the actual test result does not equal the expected result or an unexpected event (such as a loss of power) is encountered.

Testing.

Examining the behavior of a program by executing the program on sample data sets.

Third Party.

Parties not directly managed by the holder of the manufacturing and/or import authorization.

Threat.

The potential for a "threat source" to exploit (intentional) or trigger (accidental) a specific vulnerability. (NIST SP 800-33, Withdrawn: August 2018)

Threat-source.

Either (1) intent and method targeted at the intentional exploitation of a vulnerability or (2) the situation and method that may accidentally trigger a vulnerability. (NIST SP 800-33, Withdrawn: August 2018)

Timestamp.

A record mathematically linking a piece of data to a time and date.

Traceability.

The degree to which a relationship can be established between two or more products of the development process, especially products having a predecessor-successor or master-subordinate relationship to one another; e.g., the degree to which the requirements and design of a given software component match. (IEEE) (2) The degree to which each element in a software development product establishes its reason for existing; e.g., the degree to which each element in a bubble chart references the requirement that it satisfies.

Traceability Analysis.

The tracing of (1) Software Requirements Specifications requirements to system requirements in concept documentation, (2) software design descriptions to software requirements specifications and software requirements specifications to software design descriptions, (3) source code to corresponding design specifications and design specifications to source code. Analyze identified relationships for correctness, consistency, completeness, and accuracy. (IEEE)

Traceability Matrix.

A matrix that records the relationship between two or more products; e.g., a matrix that records the relationship between the requirements and the design of a given software component. (IEEE)

Training Plan.

Documentation describing the training required for an individual based on his or her job title or description.

Training Record.

Documentation (electronic or paper) of the training received by an individual that includes, but is not limited to, the individual's name or identifier; the type of training received; the date the training occurred; the trainer's name or identifier; and an indication of the effectiveness of the training (if applicable).

Transfer.

The act or process of moving records from one location to another.

True Copy Record.

An exact copy of an original record, which may be retained in the same or different format in which it was originally generated, e.g., a paper copy of a paper record, an electronic scan of a paper record, or a paper record of electronically generated data. (MHRA) (2) Accurate reproduction of the original record regardless of the technology used to create the reproduction (for example, printing, scanning, photocopying, microfilm, or microfiche). A true copy of an electronic record must contain the entire record, including all associated metadata, audit trails, and signatures, as applicable, to preserve content and meaning.

Trust.

In the network security context, trust refers to privacy (the data is not viewable by unauthorized people), integrity (the data stays in its true form), non-repudiation (the publisher cannot say they did not send it), and authentication (the publisher–and recipient–are who they say they are).

Transient Memory.

Memory that must have a constant supply of power or the stored data will be lost.

Trustworthy Computer Systems.

- Trustworthy computer systems consist of computer infrastructure, applications, and procedures that:
- are reasonably suited to performing their intended functions;
- provide a reasonably reliable level of availability, reliability and correct operation;
- are reasonably secure from intrusion and misuse; and adhere to generally accepted security principles.

Trustworthy Records.

Reliability, authenticity, integrity, and usability are the characteristics used to describe trustworthy records from a record management perspective. (NARA)

Unplanned (Emergency) Change.

An unanticipated necessary change to a validated system requiring rapid implementation.

Usable Records.

Records that can be located, retrieved, presented and interpreted.

User.

The company or group responsible for the operation of a system. (GAMP) (see also 'Regulated User'). The GxP customer, or user organization, contracting a supplier to provide a product. In the context of this document, it is, therefore, not intended to apply only to individuals who use the system and is synonymous with 'Customer'. (EU Annex 11)

User Back-up/Alternative Procedures.

Procedure which describes the steps to be taken for the continued recording and control of the raw data in the event of a computer system interruption or failure.

Unit.

A separately testable element specified in the design of a computer software element. Synonymous to component, module (IEEE).

Unit Test.

Test of a module for typographic, syntactic, and logical errors, for correct implementation of its design, and for satisfaction of its requirements.

Usability.

A useable record is one which can be located, retrieved, presented, and interpreted. (NARA)

Users.

People or processes accessing a computer system either by direct connections (i.e., via terminals) or indirect connections (i.e., prepare input data or receive output that is not reviewed for content or classification by a responsible individual).

User ID.

A sequence of characters which is recognized by the computer and which uniquely identifies one person. The UserID is the first form of identification. UserID is also known as a PIN or identification code.

Walk-through.

A static analysis technique in which a designer or programmer leads members of the development team and other interested parties through a software product, and the participants ask questions and make comments about possible errors, violation of development standards, and other problems. (IEEE)

Workflows.

The intended steps, sequencing, specifications, calculations or other processes through which a piece of work passes from initiation to completion. E.g., operational checks, authority checks, device checks, built-in checks, accuracy checks, and so on.

Validated.

It is used to indicate a status to designate that a system or software complies with applicable GMP requirements.

Validation.

Action of proving, in accordance with the principles of Good Manufacturing Practice, that any procedure, process, equipment, material, activity or system actually leads to the expected results (see also qualification). (PIC/S)

Validation Coordinator.

A person or designee responsible for coordinating the validation activities for a specific project or task.

Validation Protocol.

A written plan stating how validation will be conducted, including test parameters, product characteristics, production equipment, and decision points on what constitutes acceptable test results. (FDA)

Validation Plan.

A multidisciplinary strategy from which each phase of a validation process is planned, implemented, and documented to ensure that a facility, process, equipment, or system does what it is designed to do. May also be known as a system or software Quality Plan.

Validation Summary Report.

Documents confirming that the entire project planned activities have been completed. On acceptance of the Validation Summary Report, the user releases the system for use, possibly with a requirement that continuing monitoring should take place for a certain time. (GAMP)

Verification.

(1) The process of determining whether the products of a given phase of the SLC fulfil the requirements established during the previous phase. (2) A systematic approach to verify that manufacturing systems, acting singly or in combination, are fit for intended use, have been properly installed, and are operating correctly. This is an umbrella term that encompasses all types of approaches to assuring systems are fit for use such as qualification, commissioning and qualification, verification, system validation, or other. (ASTM 5200) (3) Confirmation by examination and provision of objective evidence that specified requirements have been fulfilled. (FDA Medical Devices) (4) In design and development, verification concerns the process of examining the result of a given activity to determine conformity with the stated requirement for that activity.

Verification (validation) of Data.

The procedures carried out to ensure that the data contained in the final report match original observations. These procedures may apply to raw data, data in case-report forms (in hard copy or electronic form), computer printouts and statistical analysis and tables. (WHO)

Virtual Private Network.

Describes the use of encryption to provide a secure telecommunication route between parties over an insecure or public network, such as the Internet.

Vulnerability.

Weakness in system security procedures, design, implementation, internal controls, and so on, that could be accidentally triggered or intentionally exploited and results in a violation of the systems' security policy. (NIST SP 800-33, Withdrawn: August 2018)

Warehouse.

A facility or location where things are stored.

Will.

This word denotes a declaration of purpose or intent by one party, not a requirement.

Work Products.

The intended result of activities or processes. (PDA)

Worst Case.

A set of conditions encompassing upper and lower processing limits and circumstances, including those within standard operating procedures, which pose the greatest chance of process or product failure when compared to ideal conditions. Such conditions do not necessarily induce product or process failure. (FDA)

Written.

In the context of electronic records, the term "written" means "recorded, or documented on media, paper, electronic or other substrate" from which data may be rendered in a human readable form. (EMA GMP Chapter 4, 2011)

APPENDIX II: ABBREVIATIONS AND/OR ACRONYMS

ABA	American Bar Association
ACE	Access-control Entry
ACL	Access Control List
ADP	Automated Data Processing
AES	Advanced Encryption Standard
AGV	Automated Guidance Vehicle
AKA	Also Known As
ALCOA	Attributable, Legible, Contemporaneous, Original and Accurate
ALCOA+	ALCOA + Complete, Consistent, Enduring and Available
ANDAs	Abbreviated New Drug Applications
ANSI	American National Standard Institute
API	Active Pharmaceutical Ingredients
ANVISA	Agencia Nacional de Vigilancia Sanitaria (Spanish) National Health Surveillance Agency (English)
ASEAN	Association of Southeast Asian Nations
ASN.1	Abstract Syntax Notation One
ASTM	American Society for Testing and Materials
BaaS	Backup as a Service

BI	Business Intelligence
BPaaS	Business Process as a Service
CA	Certification Authority
CAPA	Corrective and Preventive Actions
C-E	Cause and Effect Analyses
CEFIC	Conseil Européen des Fédérations de l'Industrie Chimique
CFDA	China Food & Drug Administration
CFR	Code of Federal Regulation
cGMP	current Good Manufacturing Practices
CIA	Confidentiality, integrity, and availability
CMC	Chemistry, Manufacturing, and Controls
CMMI	Capability, Maturity Model Integration
CNSSI	Committee on National Security Systems Instruction
CPG	US FDA Compliance Policy Guide
CPU	Central Processing Unit
CPV	Continued Process Verification
CRC	Cyclic Redundancy Check
CRL	Certificate Revocation List
CROs	Contract Research Organizations
CSV	Computer Systems Validation
DaaS	Data as a Service
DACL	Discretionary Access Control List
DCS	Distributed Control System
DES	Data Encryption Standard
DI	Data Integrity
DIQbD	Data Integrity/Quality by Design'
DM	Data Marts
DMZ	Website's Demilitarized Zone
DN	Distinguished Name
DoD	Department of Defense
DQ	Design Qualification
DRM	Device Master Record
DSA	Digital Signature Algorithm

DSM	Design Structure Matrix
DSHEA	Dietary Supplement Health and Education Act
DSS	Digital Signature Standard
DTS	Digital Time-Stamping Service
DW	Data Warehouse
EC	European Commission
ECA	European Compliance Academy
EDMS	Electronic Document Management System
EEA	European Economic Area
EEC	European Economic Community
EFS	Encrypting File System
EMA	European Medicines Agency
EMEA	European Medicines Agency
ENISA	European Union Agency for Network and Information Security
ERM	Electronic Records Management
ERP	Enterprise Resource Planning
ETL	Extract, Transform and Load
ETSI	European Telecommunications Standards Institute
EU	European Union
EVM	Earned Value Management
FAT	Factory Acceptance Test
FD&C Act	US Food Drug and Cosmetic Act.
FDA	Food and Drug Administration
FIPS	Federal Information Processing Standards
FMEA	Failure mode and Effect Analysis
FR	US Federal Register
FTP	File Transfer Protocol
GAMP	Good Automated Manufacturing Practices
GCP	Good Clinical Practices
GDP	Good Documentation Practices
GEIP	Good E-records Integrity Practices
GERM	Good Electronic Records Management
GLP	Good Laboratory Practices

GMPs	Good Manufacturing Practices
GUI	Graphical User Interface
GXP	Refers to the various good practices regulated by the regulatory authorities. These are Good Clinical Practice (GCP), Good Distribution Practice (GDP), Good Laboratory Practice (GLP), Good Manufacturing Practice (GMP), Good Pharmacovigilance Practice (GPP) and other regulated applications in context GXP can refer to one specific set of practices or to any combination of the GXP.
HMA	Heads of Medicines Agencies
HMAC	Hash Message Authentication Code
HMI	Human–Machine Interface
IaaS	Infrastructure as a Service
ICH	International Conference for Harmonization of Technical Requirements for Registration of Pharmaceuticals for Human Use
ICS	Industrial Control System
ID	Identification
I/Os	Inputs and outputs
IEC	International Electrotechnical Commission
IEEE	Institute of Electrical & Electronic Engineers
IIS	Internet Information Services
IMDRF	International Medical Device Regulators Forum
ISRS	Information storage and retrieval system
IoT	Internet of things
ISA	International Society of Automation
ISO	International Organization for Standardization
ISPE	International Society for Pharmaceutical Engineering
ISRS	Information Storage and Retrieval System
IT	Information Technology
ITIL	IT Infrastructure Library
ITSM	IT service management

JETT	Join Equipment Transition Team
KMS	Key Management Service
LAN	Local Area Network
LIMS	Laboratory Information Management System
MA	Marketing Authorization
MES	Manufacturing Execution System
MHRA	Medicines and Healthcare Products Regulatory Agency (United Kingdom medicines and medical devices regulatory agency)
MRA	Mutual Recognition Agreements
MTTR	Mean Time to Repair or Mean time to recovery
MTBF	Mean Time Between Failures
NARA	National Archives and Records Administration
NBS	National Bureau of Standards
NDAs	New Drug Applications
NEMA	National Electrical Manufacturers Association
NIST	National Institutes of Standards and Technology
NMPA	National Medical Products Association (former CFDA).
NTP	Network Time Protocol
OECD	Organization for Economic Co-operation and Development
OMCL	Official Medicines Control Laboratories
OLAs	Operational Level Agreements
OA	Orthogonal Array
OSHA	US Occupational Safety & Health Administration
OTC	Over the Counter
OTS	Off-the-Shelf
P2V	Physical to virtual
P&ID	Process and Instrumentation Drawings
PaaS	Platform as a Service
PAI	Pre-Approval Inspections
PAT	Process Analytical Tools
PDA	Parenteral Drug Association

PFD	Process Flow Diagram
PIC/S	Pharmaceutical Inspection Co-Operation Scheme http://www.picscheme.org/
PIN	Personal Identification Number
PKCS	Public-Key Cryptography Standards
PKI	Public Key Infrastructure
PLC	Programmable Logic Controller
PQ	Performance Qualification
PQS	Pharmaceutical Quality System
P&ID	Process and Instrumentation Drawing
PV	Product Verification
QA	Quality Assurance
QbD	Quality by Design
QC	Quality Control
QFD	Quality Function Deployment
QMS	Quality Management System
QP	Qualified Person
RAM	Requirements Analysis Matrix
RAM	Random Access Memory
R&D	Research and Development
RFP	Request for Proposal
RIPEMD	Race Integrity Primitives Evaluation Message Digest
RS	Requirements Specification
RTU	Remote Terminal Unit
RWG	Requirements Working Group
SaaS	Software as a Service
SACL	System Access Control List
SAG	Scientific Archivists Group
SAP	Systems, Application and Products
SAS	The Statistical Analysis System licensed by the SAS Institute, Inc.
SAT	Site Acceptance Test
SCADA	Supervisory Control and Data Acquisition
SDLC	Software Development Life Cycle

SHA-1	Secure Hash Algorithm 1
SLA	Service Level Agreement
SLC	System Lifecycle
SME	Subject Matter Experts
SIDGP	Russia Federal State Institute of Drugs and Good Practices
SIPOC	Suppliers, Inputs, Process, Outputs, Customers
SOR	System of Record
SOPs	Standard Operating Procedures
SPC	Statistical Process Control
SQA	Software Quality Assurance
SQE	Software Quality Engineering
SQL	Structured Query Language
SSA	US Social Security Administration
SSL	Secure Sockets Layer
SWEBOK	Software Engineering Body of Knowledge
TGA	Therapeutic Goods Administration
TLS	Transport Layer Security
UCs	Underpinning Contracts
UK	United Kingdom
UPS	Uninterruptable Power Supply
US	United States
US FDA	United States Food and Drugs Administration
VOC	Voice of the customer
VPN	Virtual Privates Network
WBS	Work Breakdown Structure
WAN	Wide Area Network
WL	Warning Letter
WLAN	Wireless Local Area Network
WHO	World Health Organization
XaaS	Anything as a Service

Appendix III: References

Aide-mémoire of German ZLG regarding EU GMP Annex 11nnex 11, September 2013.

Alanazi, H., Zaidan, B., Zaidan, A., Jalab, H., Shabbir, M. Al-Nabhani, Y., "New Comparative Study between DES, 3DES and AES within Nine Factors," *Journal of Computing,* Vol 2, Issue 3, March 2010, ISSN 2151-9617 (152-157)

Amy, L. T., "*Automation Systems for Control and Data Acquisition,*" ISA, 1992.

Appel, K., "*How Far Does Annex 11 Go Beyond Part 11?*" Pharmaceutical Processing, September 2011.

APV, "*The APV Guideline "Computerized Systems" based on Annex 11 of the EU-GMP Guideline*", Version 1.0, April 1996.

ASTM, E 2500 – 13 *Standard Guide for Specification, Design, and Verification of Pharmaceutical and Biopharmaceutical Manufacturing Systems and Equipment*, 2013.

Boogaard, P., Haag, T., Reid, C., Rutherford, M., Wakeham, C., "*Data Integrity,*" Pharmaceutical Engineering Special Report, March-April, 2016.

Brown, A., "Selecting Storage Media for Long-Term Preservation," *The National Archives*, DPGN-02, August 2008.

Cappucci, W., Clark, C., Goossens, T., Wyn, S., "Annex 11 Interpretation," *Pharmaceutical Engineering*, Volume 31 Number 4 (Jul/August), 2011

Carnegie Mellon University, *Software Engineering Institute, Capability Maturity Model Integration (CMMI) for Software*, Rev 3.0.

CEFIC, "*Computer Validation Guide*", API Committee of CEFIC, January 2003.

CEFIC, "*Practical Risk-based Guide for Managing Data Integrity*," March 2019 (Rev 1).

CEFIC ICH Q7, GMPs for API: "*How to Do*" Document, January 2020 (Rev 13).

Center for Technology in Government University at Albany, SUNY, "*Practical Tools for Electronic records Management and Preservation*," July 1999.

Cloud Service Alliance, "*Cloud Control Matrix*," Rev 3.0.1, July 2014.

Cloud Service Alliance, "*Security Guidance for Critical Areas of Focus in Cloud Computing*," Rev 3.0, November 2011.

Committee on National Security Systems Instruction (CNSSI), "*Glossary*," CNSSI 4009, April 2015.

Commission Directive 91/412/EEC, *Laying down the principles and guidelines of good manufacturing practice for veterinary medicinal products*, July 1991.

Commission Directive 95/46/EC of *the European Parliament and of the Council of 24 October 1995 on the protection of individuals with regard to the processing of personal data and on the free movement of such data* http://eur-lex.europa.eu/LexUriServ/LexUriServ.do?uri=CELEX:31995L0046:en:HTML

Commission Directive 2003/94/EC, *laying down the principles and guidelines of good manufacturing practice in respect of medicinal products for human use and investigational medicinal products for human use*, October 2003.

Commission Directive 2017/1572, *supplementing Directive 2001/83/EC of the European Parliament and of the Council as regards the principles and guidelines of good manufacturing practice for medicinal products for human use*, September 2017.

Council of Europe, "*Handbook on European data protection law*", December 2013.

Churchward, D., *Good Manufacturing Practice (GMP) data integrity: a new look at an old topic*, Part 1 of 3, June 2015

Churchward, D., *Good Manufacturing Practice (GMP) data integrity: a new look at an old topic*, Part 2 of 3, July 2015.

Churchward, D., *Good Manufacturing Practice (GMP) data integrity: a new look at an old topic*, Part 3 of 3, August 2015.

Churchward, D., "GMP Compliance and Data Integrity," paper presented at *the PDA/PIC's Quality and Regulations Conference*, Brussels, Belgium, June 2015.

Cuddy, B., "EMA's Guidance on Data Integrity," presented at *the Indian Pharmaceutical Alliance Annual Congress, Mumbai*, India, 23-24 February 2017.

Department of Defense (DoD) 8320.1-M-1, "*Data Standardization Procedures*," April 1998.

ECA "*Copies in the GMP Environment - True Copies*," ECA Academy, 02 June 2021, https://www.gmp-compliance.org/gmp-news/copies-in-the-gmp-environment-true-copies?utm_source=Newsletter&utm_medium=email&utm_campaign=ECA+GMP+Newsletter+-+2021+-+KW22+-+CEU

European Compliance Academy (ECA), "*Deletion of Data: Does it have to be regulated in an SOP*?" June 2019, https://www.gmp-compliance.org/gmp-news/deletion-of-data-does-it-have-to-be-regulated-in-a-sop

ECA, "*Ensuring the data integrity of cloud service providers*," https://www.it-compliance-group.org/icg_news_7259.html, August 2019.

ECA, *IT Compliance Working Group, Shared Platform and Cloud Services Implications for Information Governance and Records Management*, http://www.it-compliance-group.org/icg_downloads.html

Eglovitch, J., "*How to Remedy Data Integrity Failures: FDA's Step-by-Step Approach.*" The Golden Sheet, October 2015.

EMA/INS/GCP/454280/2010, GCP Inspectors Working Group (GCP IWG), "*Reflection paper on expectations for electronic source data and data transcribed to electronic data collection tools in clinical trials*", August 2010.

EMA, "*EMA Questions and answers: Good manufacturing practice: Data integrity,*" August 2016.

EMA, "*Reflection Paper on the Expectations for Electronic Source Documents Used in Clinical Trials,*" August 2010.

European Union Agency for Network and Information Security (ENISA), "*Cloud Security Guide for SMEs,*" April 2015.

ETSI, "*CLOUD; Cloud private-sector user recommendations,*" November 2011.

ETSI, "*Identification of Cloud user needs,*" ETSI SR 003 381 V2.1.1, February 2016.

European Compliance Academy (ECN), *GMP Data Governance and Data Integrity Guidance*, Version 2, January 2018.

European Commission (EC), "*General Data Protection Regulation (GDPR),*" January 2012 (Proposed regulation to replace EU Data Protection Directive 95/46/EC)

European Medicines Agency (EMA) - GMP/GDP compliance – "*Questions and answers: Good manufacturing practice: Annex 11 Computerised Systems,*" https://www.ema.europa.eu/en/human-regulatory/research-development/compliance/good-manufacturing-practice/guidance-good-manufacturing-practice-good-distribution-practice-questions-answers#eu-gmp-guide-annexes:-supplementary-requirements:-annex-11:-computerised-systems-section

*EU Annex III to Guidance for the Conduct of Good Clinical Practice Inspections Computer System*s, May 2008. http://ec.europa.eu/health/files/eudralex/vol-10/chap4/annex_iii_to_guidance_for_the_conduct_of_gcp_inspections_-_computer_systems_en.pdf

*EU OMLC Quality Management Guideline on Management of Documents and Record*s, January 2016.

EudraLex, *The Rules Governing Medicinal Products in the European Union*, Volume 4, "EU Guidelines to Good Manufacturing Practice, Medicinal Products for Human and Veterinary Use Part 1, Annex 11 - Computerized Systems," June 2011. http://ec.europa.eu/health/files/eudralex/vol-4/annex11_01-2011_en.pdf.

EudraLex, *The Rules Governing Medicinal Products in the European Union*, Volume 4, "EU Guidelines to Good Manufacturing Practice, Medicinal Products for Human and Veterinary Use, Annex 15 – Validation and Qualification", October 2015.

EudraLex, *The Rules Governing Medicinal Products in the European Union*, Volume 4, "EU Guidelines to Good Manufacturing Practice, Medicinal Products for Human and Veterinary Use," Annex 16 - Certification by a Qualified Person and Batch Release, 2001.

EudraLex. *The Rules Governing Medicinal Products in the European Union*, Volume 4, "EU Guidelines for Good Manufacturing Practices for Medicinal Products for Human and Veterinary Use, Annex 20 - Quality Risk Management", February 2008.

EudraLex, *The Rules Governing Medicinal Products in the European Union*, Volume 4, "EU Guidelines to Good Manufacturing Practice, Medicinal Products for Human and Veterinary Use – Glossary", February 2013.

EudraLex, *The Rule Governing Medicinal Products in the European Union*, Volume 4, EU Guidelines for Good Manufacturing Practices for Medicinal Products for Human and Veterinary Use, Part 1, Chapter 2 – Personnel", February 2014.

EudraLex, *The Rules Governing Medicinal Products in the European Union* Volume 4, Good Manufacturing Practice, Medicinal Products for Human and Veterinary Use, Chapter 3: Premises and Equipment, 2007.

EudraLex, *The Rules Governing Medicinal Products in the European Union* Volume 4, Good Manufacturing Practice, Medicinal Products for Human and Veterinary Use, Chapter 4: Documentation, June 2011.

EudraLex, *The Rules Governing Medicinal Products in the European Union* Volume 4, Good Manufacturing Practice, Medicinal Products for Human and Veterinary Use, Chapter 7: Outsourced Activities, January 2013.

EudraLex, *The Rule Governing Medicinal Products in the European Union*, Volume 4 EU Good manufacturing practice (GMP) Medicinal Products for Human and Veterinary Use, Chapter 9: Self Inspections, 2001.

EudraLex, The Rules Governing Medicinal Products in the European Union Volume 4, *Good Manufacturing Practice, Medicinal Products for Human and Veterinary Use*: Glossary, 2007.

European Agencies Agency, Questions and Answers: Good manufacturing practice, "*EU GMP guide annexes: Supplementary requirements: Annex 11: Computerised systems*", http://www.ema.europa.eu/ema/index.jsp?curl=pages/regulation/general/gmp_q_a.jsp&mid=WC0b01ac058006e06c#section8.

European Directorate for the Quality of Medicine and Healthcare, *OMCL Validation of Computerised Systems Core Documents*, May 2009. (http://www.edqm.eu/medias/fichiers/Validation_of_Computerised_Systems_Core_Document.pdf)

European Medicines Agency (EMA), "*Q&A: Good Manufacturing Practices (GMP)*," February 2011.

Federal Information Processing Standards (FIPS), Publication 11-3, "*American National Dictionary for Information Systems,*" Windrowed, July 1979.

GAMP® *Good Practice Guide: A Risk-based Approach to Compliant Electronic Records and Signatures*, 2005.

GAMP® *Good Practice Guide: Electronic Data Archiving,* 2007.

GAMP® *Good Practice Guide: Global Information Systems Control and Compliance* - Appendix 2 – Data Management Considerations, 2005.

GAMP® Good Practice Guide: IT Control and Compliance, *International Society of Pharmaceutical Engineering*, Tampa FL, 2005.

GAMP® *Good Practice Guide: Risk Based Approach to Operation of GXP Computerized Systems*, 2010.

GAMP®/ISPE, A Risk-Based Approach to Compliant GxP Computerized Systems, *International Society for Pharmaceutical Engineering* (ISPE), Fifth Edition, February 2008.

GAMP®/ISPE, "Risk Assessment for Use of Automated Systems Supporting Manufacturing Processes – Part 2 – Risk to Records," *Pharmaceutical Engineering*, Vol. 23 No. 6, November/December 2003.

GAMP®/ISPE, *Records and Data Integrity Guide*, 2017.

GAMP®/ISPE, *Risk Assessment for Use of Automated Systems Supporting Manufacturing Process – Functional Risk, Pharmaceutical Engineering*, May/Jun 2003.

George J. Grigonis, Jr., Edward J. Subak, Jr., and Michael L. Wyrick, "Validation Key Practices for Computer Systems Used in Regulated Operations," *Pharmaceutical Technology*, pages 74-98, June 1997.

GHTF, "*Implementation of risk management principles and activities within a Quality Management System*", May 2005.

GMP Journal, "*Q&As on Annex 11 (1-4) at the Computer Validation in Mannheim, Germany, in June 2011*", Issue 7, October/November 2011.

GMP Journal, "*Q&As on Annex 11 (5-11) at the Computer Validation in Mannheim, Germany, in June 2011*", Issue 8, April/May 2012.

GMP Journal, "*Q&As on Annex 11 (12-16) at the Computer Validation in Mannheim, Germany, in June 2011*", Issue 9, October/November 2012.

GOV.UK, "*The Government Data Quality Framework: guidance*," December 2020.

Graham, L., "*Compliance matters, Good laboratory practice*," Blog MHRA Inspectorate, September 2015.

Hart, S., "Data Integrity: TGA Expectations," *paper presented at the PDA conference*, Tel Aviv, Israel, July 2015.

Health Canada, "*Good Manufacturing Practices (GMP) Guidelines for Active Pharmaceutical Ingredients (APIs*"), GUI-0104, C.02.05, Interpretation #15, December 2013.

Health Canada, "*Good manufacturing practices guide for drug products, GUI-0001*," February 2018 (Version 3).

ICH Harmonized Tripartite Guideline, "*Good Manufacturing Practice Guidance for Active Pharmaceutical Ingredients, Q7*," November 2000.

ICH Harmonized Tripartite Guideline, "*Pharmaceutical Quality Systems, Q10*," June 2008.

ICH Harmonized Tripartite Guideline, "*Good Clinical Practice, E6*", Rev 2, June 2016.

ICH Harmonized Tripartite Guideline, "*Integrated Addendum to ICH Guideline GCP E6(R1)*," November 2016.

IDA Programme of the European Commission, "*Model Requirements for the Management of Electronic Records*", https://op.europa.eu/en/publication-detail/-/publication/034484f3-e6fb-4299-9676-79dc89b433e1, October 2008 (Rev 2).

IEEE, "*Guide to the Software Engineering Body of Knowledge,*" Rev 3.0, 2014.

IPEC, *Data Integrity for Pharmaceutical Grade Excipients* (April 2020)

ISO 9001:2015, "*Quality Management Systems – Requirements.*"

ISO 11799: 2003(E), "I*nformation and documentation — Document storage requirements for archive and library materials.*"

ISO 12207:1995[9], "*Information technology – Software life cycle processes.*"

ISO 13485:2012, "*Medical devices – Quality management systems – Requirements for regulatory purposes.*"

ISO 15836-1:2017, "*Information and documentation — The Dublin Core metadata element set — Part 1: Core elements.*"

ISO 8601:2004, "*Data elements and interchange formats - Information interchange - Representation of dates and times.*"

ISO 15489-1:2016(E), "*Information and documentation — Records management - Part 1: Concepts and principles.*"

[9] *Note*: The 1995 revision is not the most recent version.

ISO/IEC 1799:2005, "*Information technology — Security techniques — Code of practice for information security management*."

ISO/IEC 27001: 2013, "*Information technology— Security techniques — Information security management systems — Requirements.*"

ISPE GAMP COP *Annex 11 – Interpretation, Pharmaceutical Engineering*, July/August 2011.

ISPE GAMP Forum, "Risk Assessment for Use of Automated Systems Supporting Manufacturing Processes – Part 2 – Risk to Records," *Pharmaceutical Engineering,* Vol. 23 No. 6, November/December 2003.

ISPE, "*Regulatory Framework – EMEA*", Dr. Kate McCormick, 2009.

ISPE, "*Regulatory Framework – PIC/S and ICH*", Dr. Kate McCormick, 2009.

ISPE GAMP®: "*A Risk Approach to Compliant GxP Computerized Systems*," International Society for Pharmaceutical Engineering (ISPE), Fifth Edition, February 2008.

ISPE/PDA, "*Good Practice and Compliance for Electronic Records and Signatures. Part 1 Good Electronic Records Management (GERM).*" July 2002.

Information Security Committee American Bar Association (ABA), "*Digital Signature Guidelines*", August 1996.

IT Infrastructure Library (ITIL), "*The Official Introduction to the ITIL Service Lifecycle,*" 2007.

ITIL Service Design, Section 5.2 - *Management of Data and Information*, 2011 Edition.

Journal for GMP and Regulatory Affairs, "*Q&As on Annex 11*", Issue 8, April/May 2012.

Kane, A., the sidebar to "Designing Optimized Formulations," *Pharmaceutical Technology* (4) 2017.

López, O., "*21 CFR Part 11: Complete Guide to International Computer Validation Compliance for the Pharmaceutical Industry*," CRC, Boca Raton, Florida 1st ed., 2004.

López, O., "A Computer Data Integrity Compliance Model", *Pharmaceutical Engineering*, Vol. 35 No. 2, March/April 2015.

López, O., "A Historical View of 21 CFR 211.68," *Journal of GxP Compliance*, Vol. 15 No. 2, May 2013.

López, O., "*Analysis of FDA 2020 DI Drug GMP Observations*," Pharma Best Practices Blog., March 2021.

López, O., "*Annex 11: Progress in EU Computer Systems Guidelines*," Pharmaceutical Technology Europe, Vol. 23, No. 6 (June), 2011. http://www.pharmtech.com/pharmtech/article/articleDetail.jsp?id=725378.

López, O., "*Annex 11 and 21 CFR Part 11: Comparisons for International Compliance*," MasterCotrol, January 2012.

López, O., "*An Easy to Understand Guide to Annex 11*," Premier Validation, Cork, Ireland, 2011, http://www.askaboutvalidation.com/1938-an-easy-to-understand-guide-to-annex-11.

López, O., "CGMP E-Records Risk Assessments," *Journal of GXP Compliance*, Vol. 22, Issue 5, September 2018.

López, O., "*Comparison of Health Authorities Data Integrity Expectations*," paper presented at the 4th Annual Data Integrity Validation, Cambridge, MA, 15-16 August 2018.

López, O., "*Computer Infrastructure Qualification for FDA Regulated Industries*," PDA and DHI Publishing, LLC. 2006.

López, O., "*Computer Technologies Security Part I - Key Points in the Contained Domain*," Sue Horwood Publishing Limited, West Sussex, United Kingdom, ISBN 1-904282-17-2, 2002.

López, O., "Computer Systems Validation", *in Encyclopedia of Pharmaceutical Science and Technology*, Fourth Edition, Taylor and Francis: New York, Published online: 23 Aug 2013; 615-619.

López, O., "*Data Integrity and your E-recs During Processing*," LinkedIn, July 2017.

López, O., "Data Integrity Expectations of EU GMP Inspectors," *Pharmaceutical Engineering Europe*, Vol. 29 No. 7, July 2017.

López, O., "*Data Integrity in Pharmaceutical and Medical Devices Regulation Operations: Best Practices Guide to Electronic Records Compliance*," CRC Press, Boca Ratón, Fl., 2017.

López, O., "Data Integrity in Manufacturing Environments," in *Manufacturing Systems: Progress and Future Directions*, M. Arezki Mellal, Eds. (Nova Science Publishers, Hauppauge, NY, 1st ed., 2021).

López, O., "Defining and Managing Raw Manufacturing Data," *Pharmaceutical Technology*, Vol 21 No 6, July 2019.

López, O., "*Digital Date and Time Stamps*," LinkedIn, June 2017.

López, O., "Electronic Records Integrity in the Data Warehouse Environments," *Journal of Validation Technology*, Vol. 22 No. 2, April 2006.

López, O., "Electronic Records Lifecycle", *Journal of GxP Compliance*," Vol. 9 No. 4, December 2015.

López, O., "*Ensuring the Integrity of Electronic Health Records*," Routledge, Boca Ratón, Fl., 2021.

López, O., "E-records Vulnerabilities," *GMP Journal*, February/March 2021, pp 9-13.

López, O., "EU Annex 11 and the Integrity of Erecs", *Journal of GxP Compliance*, Volume 18 Number 2, May 2014.

López, O., "*EU Annex 11 – Changes to Computer Systems Guidelines in the EU*", LinkedIn, August 2017.

López, O., "*EU Annex 11 Guide to Computer Validation Compliance for the Worldwide Health Agency GMP*," CRC, Boca Raton, Florida 1st ed., March 2015.

López, O., "Introduction to Data Quality," *Journal of Validation Technology*, Vol. 26 No. 2, April 2020.

López, O., "Maintaining the Validated State in Computer Systems." *Journal of GxP Compliance,* Vol. 17 No. 2, August 2013.

López, O., "Maxims Electronic Records Integrity," *Pharmaceutical Technology*, Vol. 43 No. 6, June 2019.

López, O., "Overview of Technologies Supporting Security Requirements in 21 CFR Part 11 - Part I," *Pharmaceutical Technology*, February 2002.

López, O., "Overview of Technologies Supporting Security Requirements in 21 CFR Part 11 – Part II," *Pharmaceutical Technology*, March 2002.

López, O., "*Pharmaceutical and Medical Devices Manufacturing Computer Systems Validation*," CRC Press, September 2018.

López, O., "Points be considered when validating Big Data Environments," *Journal of Validation Technology,* October 2019.

López, O., "Regulations and Regulatory Guidelines of Computer Systems in Drug Manufacturing 25 Years Later," *Pharmaceutical Engineering,* Vol. 33 No. 4, July/August 2013.

López, O., "Requirements Management," *Journal of Validation Technology,* May 2013.

López, O., "Requirements for Electronic Records Contained in 21 CFR 211," *Pharmaceutical Technology,* Vol. 36, No. 7, July 208.

López, O., "Technologies Supporting Electronic Records Integrity – Part I," *GXP Journal Articles,* Vol. 21 No. 5, May 2017.

López, O., "Technologies Supporting Electronic Records Integrity Part II," *GXP Journal Articles,* Vol. 21 No. 5, September 2017.

López, O., "*The Best Practices for E-records Complianc*e," Routledge Press, Boca Ratón, Fl., 2017.

López, O., "The Importance of Computer Systems I/Os Accuracy Checks," *GxP Lifeline,* June 2012.

López, O., "Trustworthy Computer Systems", *Journal of GxP Compliance,* Vol. 19 No. 2, July 2015.

McDowall, R.D., "Comparison of FDA and EU Regulations for Audit Trails", *Scientific Computing,* January 2014.

McDowall, R.D., "Computer Validation: Do All Roads Lead to Annex 11?", *Spectroscopy* 29(12), December 2014.

McDowall, R.D., "Data Quality and Data Integrity Are the Same, Right? Wrong!," *Spectroscopy,* Vol 34 Issue 11, November 2019, pages 22-29.

McDowall, R.D., "*Ensuring Data Integrity in a Regulated Environment*", Scientific Computing, March/April 2011.

McDowall, R.D., "*Maintaining Laboratory Computer Validation - How to Conduct Periodic Reviews?*", European Compliance Academy (ECA), GMP News, April 2012, http://www.gmp-compliance.org/pa4.cgi?src=eca_new_news_print_data.htm&nr=3085.

McDowall, R.D., "*The New GMP Annex 11 and Chapter 4 is Europe's Answer to Part 11*", European Compliance Academy (ECA), GMP News, January 2011, http://www.gmp-compliance.org/eca_news_2381_6886,6885,6738,6739,6934.html.

Mell, P., and Grance, T., "*The NIST Definition of Cloud Computing*", NIST Special Publication 800-145 National Institute of Standards and Technology, Gaithersburg, Maryland 2011.

MHRA, "*GMP/GDP Consultative Committee Note of Meeting*," October 2015. (https://www.gov.uk/government/uploads/system/uploads/attachment_data/file/483846/GMP-GDP_CC_minutes_Oct_2015_FINAL.pdf)

MHRA, "*Good Manufacturing Practice (GMP) data integrity: a new look at an old topic, part 1*," June 2015. https://mhrainspectorate.blog.gov.uk/2015/06/25/good-manufacturing-practice-gmp-data-integrity-a-new-look-at-an-old-topic-part-1/

MHRA, "*Good Manufacturing Practice (GMP) data integrity: a new look at an old topic, part 2*," July 2015.

MHRA, "*Good Manufacturing Practice (GMP) data integrity: a new look at an old topic, part 3*," August 2015.

MHRA, "*Good Laboratory Practice: Guidance on Archiving*," March 2006.

MHRA, "*GxP Data Integrity Guidance and Definitions*," March 2018.

MHRA, "*MHRA Expectation Regarding Self Inspection and Data Integrity*", December 2013.

Murphy, L., "*How to make the business case for data quality & data governance Initiative*," February 2020, https://www.linkedin.com/pulse/how-make-business-case-data-quality-governance-leo-murphy/?trackingId=78vWhB34RJyL8KnY4zA29w%3D%3D

NARA, "Guidance on Managing Records in Cloud Computing Environments," *NARA Bulletin 2010-05*, September 2010.

NARA Bulletin 2015-04: *Metadata Guidance.15*836.

NARA, "*Records Management Guidance for Agencies Implementing Electronic Signature Technologies*," October 2000.

National Medical Products Association (NMPA (former CFDA)), "*Drug Data Management Practices Guidance*," December 2020.

NIST, "*An Introduction to Computer Security: The NIST Handbook*", Chapter 7, Computer Security Risk Management (Special Publication 800-12), June 2017.

NIST, "*Guidelines for Media Sanitization*," (Special Publication 800-88r1), December 2014.

NIST, "*Guide to the Processes Approach for Improving the Usability of Electronic Health Records*," NISTIR 7741, November 2010.

NIST, "*Managing Information Security Risk*," (Special Publication 800-39), March 2011.

NIST, "*Recommendation for Key Management, Part 1: General*", (Special Publication 800-57 Part 1 Rev 5), May 2020.

NIST, "*Recommendation for Key Management: Part 2 – Best Practices for Key Management Organizations*," (Special Publication 800-57 Part 2), May 2019.

NIST, "*Systems Security Engineering: Considerations for a Multidisciplinary Approach in the Engineering of Trustworthy Secure Systems*," (Special Publication 800-160 Vol 1), June 2004.

NIST, "*Underlying Technical Models for Information Technology Security*," December 2001, (Special Publication 800-33, withdrawn: August 2018).

OECD, "*Application of GLP of the Working Group on GLP*," April 2016.

OECD, "*The Application of GLP Principles to Computerized Systems*" OECD Guidance Document (Draft), September 2014.

PDA, Technical Report No. 31, "Validation and Qualification of Computerized Laboratory Data Acquisition Systems," *PDA Journal of Pharmaceutical Science and Technology*, September 1999, Vol. 53 No. 4, Section 4.5.

PDA, Technical Report No. 32, "Auditing of Supplier Providing Computer Products and Services for Regulated Pharmaceutical

Operations," *PDA Journal of Pharmaceutical Science and Technology*, Sep/Oct 2004, Release 2.0, Vol. 58 No. 5.

PI 011-3. "*Good Practices for Computerised Systems in Regulated "GXP" Environments*", Pharmaceutical Inspection Co-operation Scheme (PIC/S), September 2007.

PIC_S PI 041-1, "*Good Practice for Data Management and Integrity in Regulated GMPGDP Environments*," July 2021.

Pressman, Roger S., "*Software Engineering – A Practitioner's Approach*", McGraw Hill, 2010.

Roemer, M., "New Annex 11: Enabling Innovation," *Pharmaceutical Technology*, June 2011.

Rx-360, "*GMP Audit Manual Data Governance and Data Integrity*," March 2018.

Safe Harbor US – *EU Agreement on Meeting Directive 95/46/EC* http://www.export.gov/safeharbor/index.asp.

Sampson, K., "*Data Integrity*," Update, Issue 6, pp. 6-10 (2014). http://www.nxtbook.com/ygsreprints/FDLI/g46125_fdli_novdec2014/index.php#/0.

Scientific Archivists Group (SAG), "*A Guide to Archiving of Electronic Records*," February 2014.

Schmitt, S., "Data Integrity", *Pharmaceutical Technology*, Volume 38 Number 7, July 2014.

Schmitt, S., "*Data Integrity - FDA and Global Regulatory Guidance*", IVT, October 2014.

Russia Federal State Institute of Drugs and Good Practices (SIDGP), "*Data Integrity & Computer System Validation Guideline*," September 2018 (Draft).

Stenbraten, A., "Cost-effective Compliance: Practical Solutions for Computerised Systems," *paper presented at the ISPE Brussels Conference, GAMP – Cost Effective Compliance*, 2011-09-19/20.

Stokes, D., "*Compliant Cloud Computing – Managing the Risks*," Pharmaceutical Engineering, 33 (4) 1 - 11, 2013.

Stokes, T., "*Management's View to Controlling Computer Systems*", GMP REVIEW, Vol 10 No 2, JULY 2011.

Syncsort Editors, "*Data Integrity vs. Data Quality: How Are They Different?*" https://blog.syncsort.com/2019/01/data-quality/data-integrity-vs-data-quality-different/, January 2019.

TGA, "*Australian Code of Good Manufacturing Practice for human blood and blood components, human tissues and human cellular therapy products*," Version 1.0 April 2013.

TGA, "*Data Management and Data Integrity (DMDI)*," April 2017, https://www.tga.gov.au/data-management-and-data-integrity-dmdi

UK Government, "*The Data Lifecycle*," in the Government Data Quality Framework, https://www.gov.uk/government/publications/the-government-data-quality-framework/the-government-data-quality-framework#The-Data-Lifecycle.

US FDA, 21 CFR Part 11, "Electronic Records; Electronic Signatures; Final Rule." *Federal Register* Vol. 62, No. 54, 13429, March 1997.

US FDA 21 CFR Part 58, *Good Laboratory Practice for Non-Clinical Laboratory Studies.*

US FDA 21 CFR Part 110, *Current Good Manufacturing Practice in Manufacturing, Packing, or Holding Human Food.*

US FDA 21 CFR Part 211, *Current Good Manufacturing Practice for Finished Pharmaceuticals,* December 2007.

US FDA 21 CFR Part 312, *Investigational New Drug Application.*

US FDA 21 CFR Part 606, *Current Good Manufacturing Practice for Blood and Blood Components.*

US FDA 21 CFR Part 803, *Medical Device Reporting.*

US FDA 21 CFR 1271, *Human Cells, Tissues, and Cellular and Tissue-Based Products.*

US FDA, "*Data Integrity and Compliance with Drug CGMP, Q&A,*" December 2018.

US FDA, "*FDA PAI Compliance Program Guidance, CPG 7346.832, Compliance Program Manual*", May 2010. http://www.ipqpubs.com/wp-content/uploads/2010/05/FDA_CPGM_7346.832.pdf

US FDA, "*CPG Section 425.100 - Computerized Drug Processing; CGMP Applicability to Hardware and Software (CPG 7132a.11),*" September 1987.

US FDA, "*CPG Section 425.200 - Computerized Drug Processing; Vendor Responsibility (CPG 7132a.12),*" September 1987.

US FDA, "*CPG Section 425.300 - Computerized Drug Processing; Source Code for Process Control Application Programs (CPG 7132a.15),*" April 1987.

US FDA, "CPG Section 425.400 - Computerized Drug Processing; Input/Output Checking *(CPG 7132a.07),*" September 1987.

US FDA, "*CPG Section 425.500 Computerized Drug Processing; Identification of "Persons" on Batch Production and Control Records (CPG 7132a.08),*" September 1987.

US FDA, "*General Principles of Software Validation; Final Guidance for Industry and FDA Staff*", CDRH and CBER, January 2002.

US FDA, "*Guidance for Industry: Blood Establishment Computer System Validation in the User's Facility*", April 2013.

US FDA, "*Guidance for Industry: Computerized Systems in Clinical Investigations*", May 2007.

US FDA, "*Guidance for Industry: Contract Manufacturing Arrangements for Drugs: Quality Agreements,*" November 2016.

US FDA, "*Guidance for Industry: Electronic Records; Electronic Signatures — Scope and Application*", August 2003.

US FDA, "*Guidance for Industry: Electronic Source Data in Clinical Investigations,*" September 2013.

US FDA, "*Guidance for Industry - Process Validation: General Principles and Practices,*" January 2011.

US FDA, "*Guide to Inspection of Computerized Systems in the Food Processing Industry,*" April 2003.

Veregin, H., "*Data Quality Parameters,*" Geographical information systems, 1999.

Vibbert, J.M., "The Internet of Things: Data Protection and Data Security," *Global Environment Information Law Journal*, Volume 7 Issue 3, Spring 2016.

Wechsler, J., "*Data Integrity Key to GMP Compliance*", Pharmaceutical Technology, September 2014.

WHO. (October 2019). "*Guideline on Data Integrity*" (QAS/19.819 Draft).

WHO, Technical Report Series No. 981, Annex 2, "*WHO Guidelines on Quality Risk Management*," 2013.

WHO, Technical Report Series No. 937, Annex 4. Appendix 5, "*Validation of computerized systems*", 2006.

Wingate, G., "*Validating Automated Manufacturing and Laboratory Applications: Putting Principles into Practice*", Taylor & Francis, 1997.

Yves, S., "*ALCOA+ - what does it means?*," ECA, May 2021.

Yves, S., "*New Annex 11, Evolution and Consequences*", www.pharma-mag.com, January/February, 2012.

Appendix IV: E-Records Handling – 21 CFR Part 211 [1]

Introduction

The US FDA's introduction of regulatory requirements to computer systems can be traced back to the first publication of the GMP regulations. These requirements apply to computer systems that affect product quality and over records known to be required by existing regulations. In 1963, CFR Part 211.2(b) was incorporated as part of the first publication of the cGMP regulations. It stressed backups and documentation, including hard copies of master formulas, specifications, test records, master production and control records, and batch production records (batch production and control records), or calculations.

By 1976, the cGMP regulations combined Parts 211.2(b) and 211.68. The outcome of this combination was the updated 21 CFR Part 211.68 (Automatic, mechanical, and electronic equipment).

For all good practice disciplines regulated by competent authorities, it must be possible to reconstruct studies and reports from raw data. Electronic records may be needed to support any paper printouts [2]. Specifically, 21 CFR 211, 211.180(d) requires records to be retained "either as original records or true copies such as photocopies, microfilm, microfiche, or other accurate reproductions of the original records."

Speaking strictly on the integrity of the e-records managed by data handling systems, the applicable requirements in 211.68 [3] in 1976 were:

- The e-record must be controlled, including records retention, backup, and security.
- There must be procedural controls and technologies to ensure the accuracy and security of computer systems I/Os data.
- Data servers and associated data handling must have adequate controls to prevent unauthorized access, changes, inadvertent erasures, or loss of e-records.

The 2008 revision to 211.68(b) still maintains the above requirements.

The revision of 2008 incorporates a new section in 211.68 associated with a data integrity requirement, 211.68(c).

Based on the above requirements, the relevant principles applicable to e-records in the 2008 cGMP are [4]: Access Authorization Authorization, Data I/Os, Data Storage, Backup and Accuracy Check.

Access Authorization Authorization Principles

- Computer systems should have sufficient controls to prevent unauthorized access or changes to e-records [5].
- There should be controls to prevent omissions in e-records (e.g., the system turned off and data not captured). There should be a record of any data change made, the previous entry, who made the change, and when the change was made [6].

Data Input/Output Principles

- Input to and output from the computer or other records or data must be checked for accuracy [7].
- In the context of data integrity, computer systems must be validated to ensure accuracy, reliability, consistent intended performance, and the ability to discern invalid or altered records [8].
- Where critical data are being entered manually, there should be an additional check on the accuracy of the entry. It can be done by a second operator or by the system itself [9].
- Computer systems exchanging data electronically with other systems should include appropriate built-in checks for the correct and secure entry and processing of data to minimize the risks [5, 10].

Data Storage and Backup Principles

- A means of ensuring e-records protection should be established for all computer systems [11].
- In addition to the security-related controls, regular back-ups of all files, e-records and data entered into the computer should be made [5].
- Measures must be taken to assure that backup data are exact and complete, and secure from alteration, inadvertent erasure, and loss [6].
- There must be written procedural controls describing periodic reviews, including e-records reviews. The objective of the e-records systematic review is to confirm that they have been accurately and reliably transferred [5].
- A backup system should be provided if system breakdowns or failures would result in the permanent loss of records.

ACCURACY CHECK

The control associated with 21 CFR Part 211.68(c) is similar to the Accuracy Checks associated with EU Annex 11 p6. It establishes that there should be additional verification on the accuracy of the data entered for data entered manually. This verification can be a second person or by a validated automated system.

21 CFR Part 211.68(c) states that:

> "(c) Such automated equipment used for the performance of operations addressed by Sec. Sec. 211.101(c) or (d), 211.103, 211.182, or 211.188(b) [11] can satisfy the requirements included in those sections relating to the performance of an operation by one person and checking by another person if such equipment is used in conformity with this section, and one person checks that the equipment properly operated."

REFERENCES

[1] López, O., "*Requirements for Electronic Records Contained in 21 CFR 211*," Pharmaceutical Technology, Vol 36, No 7, July 2008.

[2] PI 011-3. "*Good Practices for ComputerizedComputerized Systems in Regulated "GXP" Environments*", Pharmaceutical Inspection Co-operation Scheme (PIC/S), September 2007.

[3] US FDA, Code of Federal Regulations, Title 21 Food and Drugs, Parts 210 and 211, Proposed Rule; *Current Good Manufacturing Practice in Manufacture, Processing, Packing, or Holding, Federal Register* Vol. 41 No. 31, 6878-6891, February 13, 1976.

[4] FDA, Code of Federal Regulations, Title 21 Food and Drugs, Parts 210 and 211, Final Rule; *Amendments to the Current Good Manufacturing Practice regulations for Finished Pharmaceuticals; Federal Register,* Vol. 73, No. 174, 51919-51933, September 8, 2008.

[5] Code of Federal Regulations, Title 21, *Food and Drugs* (Government Printing Office, Washington DC) Part 211.68(b).

[6] US Federal Register Vol 43 No 45013, September 29, 1978. US CGMP rev., comment paragraph 185.

[7] *Compliance Policy Guides associated with computer-related systems were issued by the FDA throughout the 1980s as guidelines or interpretations of the applicable CFRs.*

[8] López, O., "*A Guide to Computer Compliance Guides*," Journal of cGMP Compliance, January 1997.

[9] *US Federal Register* Vol 43 No 45013, September 29, 1978. US CGMP rev. comment paragraph 186.

[10] *US FDA Compliance Policy Guides* (CPG), Sec. 425.400 ComputerizedComputerized Drug Processing; Input/Output Checking

[11] ICH Q7, "*GMPs Guide for Active Pharmaceutical Ingredients,*" (2007).

Additional Readings

FDA, Code of Federal Regulations, Title 21 Food and Drugs, Parts 210 and 211, Final Rule; Amendments to the Current Good Manufacturing Practice regulations for Finished Pharmaceuticals; Federal Register, Vol. 73, No. 174, 51919-51933, September 8, 2008.

López, O., "*A Historical View of 21 CFR 211.68*," Journal of GxP Compliance, Volume 15, Issue 2 (Spring), 2011.

López, O., "*Requirements for Electronic Records Contained in 21 CFR 211*," Pharmaceutical Technology, Vol 36, No 7, July 2008.

Appendix V: E-Records Handling – EU Annex 11 [1]

Introduction

E-records handling may include classifying, storing, securing, and physical deletion (or, in some cases, archival preservation) of records. The ISO 15489: 2001 standard defines records handling as "The field of management responsible for the efficient and systematic control of the creation, receipt, maintenance, use and disposition of records, including the processes for capturing and maintaining evidence of and information about business activities and transactions in the form of records".

The general principles of records handling apply to records in any format. Digital records (a.k.a. electronic records or e-records) raise specific issues. It is more difficult to ensure that records' content, context, and structure is preserved and protected when the records do not have a paper-based existence.

The EU GMP requirements on data integrity for medicinal and veterinary products can be found in Article 9 item 2, Directive/ 2003/94/EC/and 91/412/EEC, respectively. Undoubtedly, the area in which most Annex 11 recommendations are made is e-records and how to manage e-records.

> *"When electronic, photographic or other data processing systems are used instead of written documents, the manufacturer shall first validate the systems by showing that the data will be appropriately stored during the anticipated period of storage. Data stored by those systems shall be made readily available in legible form and provided to the competent authorities at their request. The electronically stored data shall be protected, by methods such as duplication or backup and transfer on to another storage system, against loss or damage of data, and audit trails shall be maintained."*
>
> **Directive/2003/94/EC/Article 9-2**

EU Annex 11 [2] e-records handling guidelines can be categorized according to the e-record life cycle concept. This categorization can be used to understand the discussion about the controls necessary to ensure the authenticity and reliability of records. The life cycle (Chapter 3) can be described as creation, access, use, reuse, and physical deletion.

When writing this book, European Medicines Agency (EMA) is developing guidance on data integrity for EU GMP.

CREATION

> "4.8. If data are transferred to another data format or system, validation should include checks that data are not altered in value and/or meaning during this migration process."

The migration of e-records must be verified; there must be an additional check on the accuracy of the entry.

> "6. Accuracy Checks - For critical data entered manually, there should be an additional check on the accuracy of the data. This check may be done by a second operator or validated electronic means. The criticality and the potential consequences of erroneous or incorrectly entered data to a system should be covered by risk management."

Regulated users should define which data are to be used as raw data. As applicable, there should be special procedures for critical data entry requiring a second check. For example, the data entry and check for a manufacturing formula or the keying in of laboratory data and results from paper records. A second authorized person with logged name and identification may verify data entry with time and date via the keyboard. The inclusion and use of an audit trail (11p9) to capture the diversity of changes possibly impacting the data may facilitate this check.

When automated equipment is used as described under US FDA 21 CFR 211.68(c), featuring direct data capture linked to other databases and intelligent peripherals, the verification by a second individual is unnecessary. For example, firms may omit the second person component in weight check operations if scales are connected to a computer system performing checks on component quality control release status and proper identification of containers. The computer system must be validated, registering the raw materials identification, lot number and expiry date, and integrated with the recorded accurate weight data.

Data integrity should be ensured by suitably implemented and risk-assessed controls. Accidental input of inappropriate data, data type and/or out of range data should be prevented or result in an error message. So-called 'boundary checks' are encouraged [3].

ACCESS, USE AND REUSE

> "5. Data - Computerized systems exchanging data electronically with other systems should include appropriate built-in checks for the correct and secure entry and processing of data, to minimize the risks."

Based on the complexity and reliability of computer systems, there must be procedural controls and technologies to ensure the accuracy and security of computer system I/Os and e-records. The US FDA Compliance Policy Guide (CPG) 425.400 (formerly 7132a.07), "I/O Checking," establishes that computer I/Os are to be tested for data accuracy as part of the computer system qualification and, after the qualification, as part of the computer system's ongoing performance evaluation procedure. The use of input edits may mitigate the need for extensive I/O checks.

The objective of the I/O checks is to develop a method to prevent inaccurate data inputs and outputs. I/Os should be monitored to ensure the process remains within the established parameters. When tracking data on quality characteristics that demonstrate negative tendencies, the cause should be investigated, corrective action taken, and revalidation considered.

Edits can also makeup information and give the erroneous impression that a process is under control.

This error overrides must be documented during design.

> "7.1. Data Storage - Data should be secured by physical and electronic means against damage. Stored data should be checked for accessibility, readability and accuracy. Access to data should be ensured throughout the retention period."
>
> "7.2. Data Storage - Regular backups of all relevant data should be done. Integrity and accuracy of backup data and the ability to restore the data should be checked during validation and monitored periodically."

Computer system e-records must be controlled, covering record retention, backup and security. Computer systems must also have adequate controls to prevent unauthorized access or changes to e-records, inadvertent erasures, or loss.

Regular training in all security/backup relevant procedures to the person providing security and performing backups are crucial. The validated backup procedure, including storage facilities and media, should assure the integrity and availability of e-records and metadata of the e-records. The backup frequency depends on the computer system functions and the risk assessment of a loss of e-records.

Procedures for regular testing, including a test plan, for backup and disaster recovery, should be in place. A log of backup testing, including the date of testing and results, should be maintained, and a record of rectification of any errors should be kept. The physical security of the system should also be adequate to minimize the possibility of unauthorized access, willful or accidental damage by personnel or loss of e-records.

Before hardware and/or software are exchanged, a change control mechanism should be used to check that the e-records concerned can also be managed in the new configuration. If the impact assessment demonstrates that changes in the hardware and/or software mean that the stored e-records cannot be managed in the new configuration, one of the following procedures should be applied:

- the e-records in the format concerned should be converted into a form that can be printed in the new configuration;
- the components of the old hardware and/or software configuration required for printing should be retained. In this case, it should be guaranteed that a suitable alternative system is available in case the controlled system fails;
- the e-record is transferred to another medium.

The electronically stored e-records should be checked regularly for availability and integrity. Appropriate controls for electronic documents such as templates, forms and master documents should be implemented. Appropriate controls should be in place to ensure the integrity of the record throughout the retention period.

Additional references associated with this principle can be found at: Article 9 Section 2, Commission Directives 2003/94/EC; PIC/S PI 011-3; EudraLex - Volume 4 Good manufacturing practice (GMP) Guidelines, Part I – Basic Requirements for Medicinal Products, Chapter 4 – Documentation; and US FDA 21 CFR 211.68 and 21 CFR Part 11.10(c); 11.10(d); 11.10(e); 11.10(g); 11.10(h); 11.30.

> "9. Audit Trails - Consideration should be given, based on a risk assessment, to build into the system the creation of a record of all GMP-relevant changes and deletions (a system-generated "audit trail"). The

> reason should be documented for the change or deletion of GMP-relevant data. Audit trails need to be available and convertible to a generally intelligible form and regularly reviewed."

Audit trails are control mechanisms generated by computer systems that allow all raw data entered and further processed by the system to be traced back to the raw data. If the e-record needs to be changed, a second person should approve these changes and the reasons. The audit trail records should be reviewed regularly.

The date and time of the audit trail must be synchronized to a trusted date and time service.

One of the essential controls for audit trails is the link of the e-record with the associated audit trail. Audit trails can be part of the record that has been modified or a standalone record linked to the modified record. Audit trails cannot be altered. The access rights for audit trial information must be limited to print and/or read-only. The combination of authentication, digital certificates, encryption and access control lists provides the technical mechanisms needed to control the access to audit trail files.

> "12.4. Management systems for data and documents should be designed to record the identity of operators entering, changing, confirming or deleting data including date and time."

Computer systems must have adequate controls to prevent unauthorized access or changes to e-record, inadvertent erasures or loss. Procedures should ensure that:

- Access rights for all operators are clearly defined and controlled, including physical and logical access.
- Basic rules exist and are documented to ensure security related to personal passwords or passcards and related system/e-records security requirements are not reduced or negated.

- Proper authority and responsibilities are assigned to the correct organizational level.
- Identification code and password issuance are periodically checked, recalled or revised.
- Loss management exists to electronically invalidate lost, stolen or potentially compromised passwords. The system should be capable of enforcing regular changes of passwords.
- Procedures identify prohibited passwords.
- An audit log of password security breaches should be kept, and measures should be in place to address such breaches.
- The system should enforce access revocation after a specified number of unsuccessful login attempts.
- Validated recovery of original information and e-records following backup, media transfer, transcription, archiving, or system failure.
- Attempted breaches of security safeguards should be recorded and investigated.

Some equipment, such as standalone computer systems and dedicated operator equipment interfaces and instruments, may lack logical (e.g., password.) capabilities. These should be listed, justified and subjected to procedural controls.

> "17. Archiving - Data may be archived. This data should be checked for accessibility, readability and integrity. If relevant changes are to be made to the system (e.g. computer equipment or programs), then the ability to retrieve the data should be ensured and tested."

The archived records need to be trustworthy, reliable, and accessible, no matter where they are stored. The party having primary responsibility for record retention under the predicate regulations would be the party responsible for the adequacy of archiving these e-records.

PHYSICAL DELETION

The only activity not explicitly covered in Annex 11 is the computer systems and e-records retirement. The retirement of computer systems and e-records is covered implicitly as part of 11 p10. Retirement is considered a change of state of the computer, from active to inactive.

In the context of the computer system retirement and deletion of e-records:

- Suppose the e-records are transferred to another e-records format or system. In that case, validation should include checks that e-records are not altered in value and/or meaning during this migration process (11 p4.8).
- If the e-records are transferred to another system, the ability to retrieve the e-records should be ensured and tested (11 p7).

CONTROLS BASED ON SYSTEM LIFE CYCLE

The following are a set of controls that should be in place to protect the e-records. These controls are compiled based on the Annex 11 computer system lifecycle (SLC) phase [4].

Table 1. Controls based on SLC phase

Computer SLC Phase	Records Life Cycle [5]	E-records Controls
General Phase – Requirements	Analysis	1. Identify the relevant critical records. Critical records are identified in the risk analysis course (11 p1). 2. Identify data and e-records integrity-related controls based on a risk assessment. Manage the controls to mitigate the risks through the SLC (11 p1). 3. If data are transferred to another data format, identify the new format. (11 p4.8 and 11 p8.1) and control requirements (11 p5).
General Phase – Requirements	Analysis	4. Identify interfaces (11 p5) and enter the data manually (11 p6). 5. Based on risk assessment, assess the need for audit trails (11 p12.4) and controls to prevent unauthorized access to the application and the operating systems (11 p7.1, 11 p12 and 21 CFR 11.10(g)). 6. The requirements document must include a requirement(s) uncovered during the assessments of the risks. 7. Design the reports (11 p8.1), accuracy checks (11 p6), operational system checks (21 CFR Part 11.10(f)), authority checks (21 CFR Part 11.10(g)) and device checks (21 CFR Part 11.10(h)). 8. Time stamping controls. It should be utilized as a time-stamping service. If the local clock is used, the periodic coordination between the service and the local computer clock is expected. Limit the access of the computer date and time local function. Users must not access the local computer date and time function.

Table 1. (Continued)

Computer SLC Phase	Records Life Cycle [5]	E-records Controls
Project Phase – Specification, Design, Programming, Testing, Installation	Analysis	1. As part of the application qualification and associated controls, test the backup and restoration procedure(s) and verify the output of the backup (11 p7.2). Each backup set should be checked to ensure that it is error-free. 2. Verify audit trail capabilities, as applicable (11 p7.1). 3. Verify the accuracy of reports and audit trail reports (11 p8). 4. As applicable and based on the operational sequencing, test accuracy of e-records (11 p7.1). 5. If e-records are transferred to another format, the qualification must include checks that e-records new format is not altered/or meaningful during the migration process. (11 p4.8) 6. IT infrastructure must be qualified to ensure security and e-records integrity. (Principle b)
Operational and Maintenance Phases	Creation, Access, Use and Reuse, Archiving, Transfer, Archiving or Destruction	1. A means of ensuring e-records protection must be established for all computer systems (Health Canada GMP Guidelines for API (GUI-0104) Dec 2013, ICH Q7 Aug 2001, EU Annex 11 p4.8, 11 p5, 11 p6, 11 p7, 11 p8.1, 11 p12). 2. Written procedures must be available for the operation and maintenance of computer systems[10]. Management of records, Performance monitoring (11 p11), change control program (11 p10) and e-records security (11 p12), calibration and maintenance (11 p10), personnel training (11 p2), emergency recovery (11 p16), management of incidents (11 p17), e-records entry (11 p6) and modifications (WHO 4.2) and periodic re-evaluation (11 p11) are some of the procedures impacting e-records integrity. 3. The procedures and records about the security of the system and the e-records are essential and must be based on the IT policies of the regulated user and in conformance with the relevant regulatory requirements (11 p12.1).

Computer SLC Phase	Records Life Cycle [5]	E-records Controls
		4. There should be written procedures for recovery of the system following a breakdown; these procedures should include documentation and record requirements to assure retrieval and maintenance of GxP information 11 p16).-records must be secured by physical and electronic means against damage, including unauthorized access and changes to e-records (11 p12). As part of physical security must be considered security to devices used to store programs, such as tapes, disks, and magnetic strip cards. Access to these devices should be controlled. 5. Periodic (or continuous) reviews must be performed after the initial validation (11 p11). As part of a periodic review: verify stored, backup and archived e-records for accessibility, readability and accuracy; verify the output of the backup; accuracy of audit trail. As applicable, verify accurate and reliable e-records transfer (WHO 3.2). 6. Access to e-records should be ensured throughout the retention period (11 p7.1). 7. The electronically stored e-records should be checked regularly for availability and integrity (11 p7.1). 8. Following changes to the system, change control should ensure the availability and integrity of the e-records on the backup copies by restoring the e-records on a trial basis (11 p10 and 11 p7.2). 9. E-record errors, complete loss in data, and data integrity must be reported and investigated. Corrective action(s) must be taken following the investigation (11 p13). The GMP regulators expect any resulting recommendations to be implemented as soon as reasonably practical. 10. When applicable, there must be controls to prevent the system turned off and e-records not being captured (11 p5). 11. For critical records entered or e-records amended (WHO 4.2) manually, there should be an additional check on the accuracy of the data and only entered by persons authorized to do so (11 p6).

Table 1. (Continued)

Computer SLC Phase	Records Life Cycle [5]	E-records Controls
		12. Where an e-record is deleted before meeting its approved retention, an audit trail of the deletion is required until the end of the approved retention period (11 p7.1). When outside agencies are used to providing computer service, there should be a formal agreement including a clear statement of the responsibilities of that outside agency (11 p3.1).
Retirement Phase	E-record Destruction	1. In the context of the computer system retirement: • suppose the e-records are transferred to another e-records format or system. In that case, validation should include checks that e-records are not altered in value and/or meaning during this migration process (11 p4.8). • If the e-records are transferred to another system, the ability to retrieve the e-records should be ensured and tested (11 p7).

References

[1] López, O., "Annex 11: Progress in EU Computer Systems Guidelines," *Pharmaceutical Technology Europe*, Vol. 23, No. 6 (June), 2011.

[2] EudraLex Volume 4, "*EU Guidelines to Good Manufacturing Practice, Medicinal Products for Human and Veterinary Use, Annex 11 - Computerized Systems*," June 2011. http://ec.europa.eu/health/files/eudralex/vol-4/annex11_01-2011_en.pdf.

[3] European Medicines Agency (EMA) - GMP/GDP compliance – "*Questions and answers: Good manufacturing practice: Annex 11 Computerised Systems Question 2,*" http://www.ema.europa.eu/ema/index.jsp?curl=pages/regulation/q_and_a/q_and_a_detail_000027.jsp&mid=WC0b01ac05800296ca#section9.

[4] *Lifecycle - All phases in the system's life from initial requirements until retirement, including design, specification, programming, testing, installation, operation, and maintenance.* (EU Annex 11).

[5] López, O. "Maintaining the Validated State in Computer Systems", *Journal of GXP Compliance*. Volume 17 Number 2, August 2013 (http://www.ivtnetwork.com/article/maintaining-validated-state-computer-systems).

Additional Readings

Heddell, G., "*Data Integrity: An EU Perspective*," paper presented at the Third Annual ISPE-FDA CMP Conference, Baltimore, Maryland, 2-4 June 2014.

López, O., "*Annex 11 and Electronic Records Integrity*," in EU Annex 11 Guide to Computer Validation Compliance for the Worldwide Health Agency GMP, Eds. (CRC Press, Boca Raton, Fl, 1st ed., March 2015), pp. 229-251.

Appendix VI: Regulatory Analysis

Crosswalk between EU Annex 11 and US FDA – 211, 820, 11; other guidelines and regulations. Orlando López – Rev09Sep20. https://drive.google.com/drive/folders/1EqeWvGAipuuwQJh2qf0v7ru50BiWzov-?usp=sharing

	References				
	Old Annex 11	**211**	**820**	**11**	**Others/Guidelines**
Principle.					GAMP 5 –Management Appendix M3. Data quality element: Accurate.
This annex applies to all forms of computerised systems used as part of a GMP regulated activities. A computerised system is a set of software and hardware components which together fulfill certain functionalities.		211.68[11]	820.70(i).	11.2(b).	EU Directives 2017/1572 and 91/412/EEC. PIC/S PI 011-3. ISO 13485 7.5.2. Article 1 draft Annex 2 CFDA GMP. OECD Guidance Document, Section 1.1.1. 211.68(a)

[11] O. López, "*A Historical View of 21 CFR Part 211.68*", Journal of GXP Compliance, Vol. 15 No. 2, Spring 2011.

Regulatory Analysis: (Continued)

	References				
	Old Annex 11	**211**	**820**	**11**	**Others/Guidelines**
The application should be validated; IT infrastructure should be qualified.	11-3	211.68	820.70(i). 820.30(g) 820.170	11.10(a).	Eudralex Volume IV, Glossary PIC/S PI 011-3. ICH Q7A Good Manufacturing Practice Guidance for Active Pharmaceutical Ingredients, Sections 5.40 and 5.41. WHO - Technical Report Series, No. 937, 2006. Annex 4. Appendix 5, Section 7.1 (Hardware). ISO 13485 7.5.2; 7.3.6; 7.2; 7.2.1; 7.2.2 Article 10 draft Annex 2 CFDA GMP. GAMP GPG: IT Infrastructure Control and Compliance, 2005. OECD Guidance Document, Section 1.1.2. ICH E6 Guideline for GCP (June 1996), Section 5.5.3(a) ANMAT (Argentina) 5.21 US FDA General Principles of Software Validation, Section 5.2.6. Part II - Basic Requirements for Active Substances used as Starting Materials, Section 5.40. Sections 8.1 and 9.10 Russian Federation DI Guideline Health Canada GMP Guidelines C.02.05 – 8.f.i.

	References				
	Old Annex 11	**211**	**820**	**11**	**Others/Guidelines**
General.					
Where a computerised system replaces a manual operation, there should be no resultant decrease in product quality, process control or quality assurance. There should be no increase in the overall risk of the process.	Principle				PIC/S PI 011-3. US FDA CPG 7348.810 - Sponsors, CROs, and Monitors. Thailand CSV GMPs. Article 2 draft Annex 2 CFDA GMP.

Regulatory Analysis: (Continued)

	References				
	Old Annex 11	211	820	11	Others/Guidelines
1. Risk Management. Risk management should be applied throughout the lifecycle of the computerised system considering patient safety, *data integrity* and product quality. As part of a risk management system, decisions on the extent of validation and *data integrity controls* should be based on a justified and documented risk assessment of the computerised system.		211.68(b)[12]	820.30(g)		812.66[13] ICH Q9 Quality Risk Management. ICH Q7 5.40 ICH E6 (R2) 5.0.2 ICH E6 (R2) 1.65 NIST, Risk Management Guide for Information Technology Systems, Special Publication 800- 30. GHTF, Implementation of risk management principles and activities within a Quality Management System. ISO 14971:2007, Medical devices – Application of risk management to medical devices GAMP Forum, Risk Assessment for Use of Automated Systems Supporting Manufacturing Process – Risk to Record, Pharmaceutical Engineering, Nov/Dec 2002. GAMP/ISPE, Risk Assessment for Use of Automated Systems Supporting Manufacturing Process – Functional Risk, Pharmaceutical Engineering, May/Jun 2003. EU Annex 20. US FDA Guidance for the Content of Pre-Market Submission for

[12] Federal Register, Vol 60 No. 13, 4087-4091, January 20, 1995.

[13] All 21 CFR Part 812 regulations apply equally to both paper records and electronic records. The use of computer systems in clinical investigations does not exempt IDEs from any Part 812 regulatory requirement.

	References				
	Old Annex 11	**211**	**820**	**11**	**Others/Guidelines**
1. Risk Management.					Software Contained in Medical Devices, May 2005. Pressman, Roger S., Software Engineering – A Practitioner's Approach, McGraw Hill. GAMP 5 –Management Appendices M3 and M4; Operational Appendices O2, O6, O8, O9. ISO 13485 7.3.6 WHO, Technical Report Series No. 281, 2013. Health Canada API, C.02.05, Interpretation #12. Articles 3. 6, 12 draft Annex 2 CFDA GMP. OECD Guidance Document, Section 1.2. ANMAT (Argentina) 5.21 US FDA General Principles of Software Validation Section 4.8 PIC/S Guidance PI 011-3, Sections 4.5 and 4.6. Establishing data criticality and inherent integrity risk, MHRA March 2018, March 2018). Section 5.3 PIC/S PI 041-1 (Draft3). Section 5.0, WHO, Technical Report Series No. 995, 2016. Sections 6.2 and 9.2 Russian Federation DI Guideline Sections 4.7 and 5 in WHO QAS19_819. CEFIC DI Best Practices Guide for API (FINAL March 2019) Guide to CSV, Anvisa Sections 4.1.4, 6.0 DI OECD, Sections 5.4 and 5.5

Regulatory Analysis: (Continued)

	References				
	Old Annex 11	**211**	**820**	**11**	**Others/Guidelines**
2. Personnel. There should be close cooperation between all relevant personnel such as Process Owner, System Owner, Qualified Persons and IT. All personnel should have appropriate qualifications, level of access and defined responsibilities to carry out their assigned duties. (Data quality element: Attributable)	11-1	211.101(d), 211.122, 211.186, 211.188(b) (11)	820.20(b) (1) and (2); 820.25	11.10(i) 11.10(j) 11.100(b)	EudraLex, The Rule Governing Medicinal Products in the European Union, Volume 4, EU Guidelines for Good Manufacturing Practices for Medicinal Products for Human and Veterinary Use, Part 1, Chapter 2 – Personnel, February 2014 21 CFR 110(c). 21 CFR 606.160(b)(5)(v). 21 CFR Part 312.53(a) and .53(d). 21 CFR 58.29 WHO - Technical Report Series, No. 937, 2006. Annex 4, Section 13 GAMP 5 6.2.3.1, 6.2.3.3, 6.2.3.3. 6.2.3.5 and Operational Appendix O12. ISO 13485 5.5; 5.5.1; 5.5.3; 6.2; 6.2.1; 6.2.2 Japan CSV Guideline (Guideline on Management of Computerized Systems for Marketing Authorization Holder and Manufacturing of Drugs and Quasi-drugs, October 2010), Section 6.8. Thailand CSV GMPs, Clause 510. Health Canada API, C.02.006 OECD Guidance Document, Section 1.3. Brazil API (RDC Resolution #69 Chapter VI Section VI Art. 258)) US FDA Data Integrity (Draft) Guidance III.16 Section 8.0, WHO, Technical Report Series No. 995, 2016. Section 6.4.3 Russian Federation DI Guideline DI NMPA (former CFDA) Article 10

	References				
	Old Annex 11	211	820	11	Others/Guidelines
3. Suppliers and Service Providers. 3.1 When third parties (e.g., suppliers, service providers) are used e.g., to provide, install, configure, integrate, validate, maintain (e.g., via remote access), modify or retain a computerised system or related service or for data processing, formal agreements must exist between the manufacturer and any third parties, and these agreements should include clear statements of the responsibilities of the third party. IT-departments should be considered analogous.	11-18	Sub Part B 211.34	820.20(b) (1) and (2), 820.50		EudraLex, The Rules Governing Medicinal Products in the European Union Volume 4, Good Manufacturing Practice, Medicinal Products for Human and Veterinary Use, Chapter 7: Outsourced Activities, January 2013. 21 CFR 110(c). ICH Q7 Good Manufacturing Practice Guidance for Active Pharmaceutical Ingredients ICH Q10 Section 2.7 Management of Outsourced Activities and Purchased Materials. WHO - Technical Report Series, No. 937, 2006. Annex 4. Appendix 5, Section 6.2. GAMP 5 Section 6.1.4. GAMP 5 –Management Appendices M2 and M6. ISO 13485 5.5; 5.5.1; 5.5.3; 6.2; 6.2.1; 6.2.2' 7.4; 7.4.1. China GMPs, Section 7. Thailand CSV GMPs, Clause 527. PDA, Technical Report No. 32 Auditing of Supplier Providing Computer Products and Services for Regulated Pharmaceutical Operations, PDA Journal of Pharmaceutical Science and Technology, Sep/Oct 2004, Release 2.0, Vol 58 No 5. CEFIC CSV Guide, Section 7.4.6. Article 4 draft Annex 2 CFDA GMP. OECD Guidance Document, Section 1.6.

Regulatory Analysis: (Continued)

	References				
	Old Annex 11	**211**	**820**	**11**	**Others/Guidelines**
3. Suppliers and Service Providers. 3.2 The competence and reliability of a supplier are key factors when selecting a product or service provider. The need for an audit should be based on a risk assessment. 3.3 Documentation supplied with commercial off-the-shelf products should be reviewed by regulated users to check that user requirements are fulfilled.					PIC/S Guidance PI 011-3 Sections 5.1, 5.2, 11. Section 6.20, MHRA March 2018. Section 10.0, PIC/S PI 041-1 (Draft3). Section 7.0, WHO, Technical Report Series No. 995, 2016. Section 9.3 Russian Federation DI Guideline Section 7, WHO QAS19_819 Guide to CSV, Anvisa Section 4.1.5 DI NMPA (former CFDA) Article 11

	References				
	Old Annex 11	**211**	**820**	**11**	**Others/Guidelines**
3. Suppliers and Service Providers. 3.4 Quality system and audit information relating to suppliers or developers of software and implemented systems should be made available to inspectors on request. 3.5 The supplier should be assessed appropriately.					

Regulatory Analysis: (Continued)

	References				
	Old Annex 11	211	820	11	Others/Guidelines
Project Phase.					OECD Guidance Document, Section 2
4. Validation. 4.1 The validation documentation and reports should cover the relevant steps of the life cycle. Manufacturers should be able to justify their standards, protocols, acceptance criteria, procedures and records based on their risk assessment. 4.2 Validation documentation should include change control records (if applicable) and reports on any deviations observed during the validation process.	11-2; 11-4; 11-5; 11-7	211.68; 211.100(a), (b).	820.3(z), 803.17 820.40 820.170 820.30(g), 820.70(g) 820.70(i). 820.70(i) 820.30(c); 820.3(z) and (aa); 820.30(f) and (g)	11.10(a); 11.10(k); 11.10(h); 11.300(e)	EU Directives 2017/1572, Article 9 Section 2. ISO 90003:2004, Sections 7.3.2; 7.3.3; 7.3.4; 7.3.5; 7.3.6.2a; 7.3.6.2.b; 7.3.6.2.c; 7.5.1.5; 7.5.1.6; 7.3.6.2d; 7.3.7; 7.5.3.2 ISO-27000, Sections 12.1, 12.2 Medicines and Healthcare products Regulatory Agency (MHRA) (UK). IEEE. PIC/S PI 011-3 Sections 6.3, 7, 9, 10, 13.2, 14.3, 23.8, 23.10 21 CFR 606.160(b)(5)(ii) and 606.100(b)(15). ICH Q7 Good Manufacturing Practice Guidance for Active Pharmaceutical Ingredients, Sections 5.41, 12.2. ICH Q9 Quality Risk Management. 11-1 21 CFR 58.61; 63(a) and (c); 58.81(c) and (d); 58.33 21 CFR 59.190 Blood Establishment Computer System Validation in the User's Facility, April 2013. US FDA General Principles of Software Validation. WHO - Technical Report Series, No. 937, 2006. Annex 4. Appendix 5 GAMP 5 Sections 4.2.1, 4.2.3, 4.2.4, 5.2.3, 5.2.5, 6.1.5, 6.1.6, 6.2.6, 6.2.8, 6.2.9, 6.2.10 GAMP 5 Development Appendices: D1 – D7; Management Appendices M1 – M10; Operational Appendix O1 21 CFR 1271.160(d)

	References				
	Old Annex 11	**211**	**820**	**11**	**Others/Guidelines**
4. Validation. 4.3 An up to date listing of all relevant systems and their GMP functionality (inventory) should be available. For critical systems an up to date system description detailing the physical and logical arrangements, data flows and interfaces with other systems or processes, any hardware and software pre-requisites, and security measures should be available.			820.30 820.50		21 CFR 803.17; 21 CFR 803.18 EU Annex 15. Brazilian Medical Devices (RDC No 16) Sections 1.2.4, 4.1.8, 4.2.1.1, 5.4.6, 5.5.2 and 5.5.3, 5.6. ISO 13485 2.3; 7.2; 7.2.1; 7.2.2; 7.5.1.2.2; 7.3.6; 6.3; 7.5.2. ISO/TR 14969:2004 7.5.2 ISO 27000 Section 7.1 Japan CSV Guideline (Guideline on Management of Computerized Systems for Marketing Authorization Holder and Manufacturing of Drugs and Quasi- drugs, October 2010), Sections 4, 5 and 9. China GMPs Article 109. Thailand CSV GMPs, Clauses 511, 512, 513, 514, 516. Health Canada API, C.02.05 Interpretation #12; #13; #14; 17. C.02.015 Interpretation #3; #13.5 Articles 5, 7, 8, 9, 11, 13 draft Annex 2 CFDA GMP. OECD Guidance Document, Sections 1.5., 1.7, 1.9, 2.1, 2.3, 2.4, 2.5, 2.6, 2.7, 2.8 ANMAT (Argentina) 5.25

Regulatory Analysis: (Continued)

	References				
	Old Annex 11	**211**	**820**	**11**	**Others/Guidelines**
4. Validation. 4.4 User Requirements Specifications should describe the required functions of the computerised system and be based on documented risk assessment and GMP impact. User requirements should be traceable throughout the life cycle[14]. 4.5 The regulated user should take all reasonable steps, to ensure that the system has been developed in accordance with an appropriate quality management system. The supplier should be assessed appropriately.					US FDA General Principles of Software Validation 4.1, 4.5, 5.1, 5.2, 5.2.1, 5.2.2, 5.2.3, 5.2.4, 5.2.5, 5.2.6, 23.10 Brazil API (RDC Resolution #69 Chapter VI Section VI) WHO Technical Report 986 Annex 2 (Section 15.9) ITIL Service Design (Section 5.2.8) US FDA Data Integrity (Draft) Guidance III.3 Part II - Basic Requirements for Active Substances used as Starting Materials, Section 5.41 and 5.42. Sections 5, 6.8, 6.11, 6.17.1, 6.19 and 5, MHRA March 2018. Section 9.0, WHO, Technical Report Series No. 995, 2016. NSF 363-14 Section 6.3.2.3 (a) and (c) OMCL 7.3 Sections 8.2.4 and 9.2 Russian Federation DI Guideline Sections 9.4, 9.5, 9.6, and 9.7 Russian Federation DI Guideline Section 11, WHO QAS19_819. Section 9.2, PIC/S PI 041-1 (Draft3). Guide to CSV, Anvisa Sections 4.1.3, 5.0, 8.0, 9.0, 10.0, 12.0. DI OECD Sections 6.0, 7.10 DI NMPA (former CFDA) Chapter IV

[14] O. López, "*Requirements Management*", Journal of Validation Technology, Vol. 17 No. 2, Spring 2011.

	References				
	Old Annex 11	**211**	**820**	**11**	**Others/Guidelines**
4. Validation. 4.6 For the validation of bespoke or customised computerised systems there should be a process in place that ensures the formal assessment and reporting of quality and performance measures for all the life-cycle stages of the system formal assessment and reporting of quality and performance measures for all the life-cycle stages of the system.					

Regulatory Analysis: (Continued)

	References				
	Old Annex 11	**211**	**820**	**11**	**Others/Guidelines**
4. Validation. 4.7 Evidence of appropriate test methods[15] and test scenarios should be demonstrated. *Particularly, system (process) parameter limits, data limits and error handling should be considered*[16]. Automated testing tools and test environments should have documented assessments for their adequacy.					

[15] Test methods – With the Black-Box Test, the test cases are derived solely from the description of the test object, the inner structure of the object is thus not considered when creating the test plan; With the White-Box Test the test cases are derived solely from the structure of the test object; With the Source-Code Review the source code is checked against the documentation describing the system by one or several professionals. The APV Guideline ÓComputerized SystemsÓ based on Annex 11 of the EU-GMP Guideline, April 1996.

[16] This sentence is related with the additional checks covered in Accuracy Checks (11-6).

	References				
	Old Annex 11	**211**	**820**	**11**	**Others/Guidelines**
4. Validation. 4.8 *If data are transferred to another data format or system, validation should include checks that data are not altered in value and/or meaning during this migration process*[17].					
Operational Phase.					GAMP 5 –Operational Appendix O12. OECD Guidance, Section 3. ANMAT (Argentina) 5.22 and 5.23 Part II - Basic Requirements for Active Substances used as Starting Materials, Section 5.44. Guide to CSV, Anvisa Section 11.0

[17] Annex 11-4.8 is complemented with 11-7.1.

Regulatory Analysis: (Continued)

	References				
	Old Annex 11	**211**	**820**	**11**	**Others/Guidelines**
5. Data. Computerised systems exchanging data electronically with other systems should include appropriate built-in checks for the correct and secure entry and processing of data, in order to minimize the risks.[18] (Data quality element: Accurate)	11-6	211.68(b). 211.88. 211.194(d)	806.1 820.25 820.70 (a) 820.180 820.184	11.10(a); 11.10(b); 11.10(e); 11.10(f); 11.10(g); 11.10(h); 11.30.	US FDA 425.400; 803.1; 803.10; 803.14; 806.10; 806.30; 58.15; 58.33; 58.35; 59.190 EudraLex - Volume 4 Good manufacturing practice (GMP) Guidelines, Part I – Basic Requirements for Medicinal Products, Chapter 4 – Documentation. EU Directives 2017/1572, Chapter 9, Article 2. GAMP 5 –Operational Appendix O9. Thailand CSV GMPs, Clause 515. OECD Guidance, Section 2.9. ICH Q7 Section 5.45. ITIL, Service Design (Chapter 5.2.10) Section 9.2.1 (Data transfer between systems) and 9.5, PIC/S PI 041-1 (Draft). Section 6.7, MHRA March 2018 Section 12.13, WHO QAS19_819 PIC/S PI 041-1 (Draft3), Section 9.5-1. DI OECD Section 7.9 DI NMPA (former CFDA) Article 26 item (2).

[18] Annex 11-5 is fundamental in erecs integrity and it is related with Annex 11-4.7.

	References				
	Old Annex 11	**211**	**820**	**11**	**Others/Guidelines**
6. Accuracy Checks. For critical data[19] entered manually, there should be an additional check on the accuracy of the data. This check may be done by a second operator or by validated electronic means. The criticality and the potential consequences of erroneous or incorrectly entered data to a system should be covered by risk management.[20] (Data quality element: Accurate)	11-9	211.68(c).	820.25 820.70	11.10(f)	The APV Guideline "Computerized Systems" based on Annex 11 of the EU-GMP Guideline. EudraLex - Volume 4 Good manufacturing practice (GMP) Guidelines, Part I - Basic Requirements for Medicinal Products, Chapter 4 – Documentation. PIC/S PI 011-3. EU Annex 11-1. WHO - Technical Report Series, No. 937, 2006. Annex 4. Appendix 5, Section 4.5. ISO 13485 6.2; 6.2.1; 6.2.2; 7.5. Thailand CSV GMPs, Clause 518. Health Canada API, C.02.015 Interpretation #18. Article 15 draft Annex 2 CFDA GMP. OECD Guidance, Section 3.1. ANMAT (Argentina) 5.26 and 5.30 ITIL, Service Design (Chapter 5.2.10) Part II - Basic Requirements for Active Substances used as Starting Materials, Sections 5.45 and 5.49. OMC 7.3 Section 6.11.1, MHRA March 2018 Section 8.1.1 Russian Federation DI Guideline

[19] The term "critical data" in this context is interpreted as meaning data with high risk to product quality or patient safety. ISPE GAMP COP Annex 11 – Interpretation, July/August 2011.

[20] Annex 11-6 is another fundamental section related with erecs integrity.

Regulatory Analysis: (Continued)

	References				
	Old Annex 11	211	820	11	Others/Guidelines
6. Accuracy Checks.					Section 9.4, WHO QAS19_819 PIC/S PI 041-1 (Draft3), Section 9.5-1. DI NMPA (former CFDA) Article 26 item (1).
7. Data Storage. 7.1 Data should be secured by both physical and electronic means against damage. Stored data should be checked for accessibility, readability and accuracy. Access to data should be ensured throughout the retention period. (Data quality element: Legible)	11-13 11-14	211.68(b). 211.180(e).	803.1 820.20 820.40 820.180 806.1	11.10(c) 11.10(d) 11.10(e) 11.10(g) 11.10(h) 11.30.	812.38. EU Directives 2017/1572, Article 9 Section 2. PIC/S PI 011-3. EudraLex - Volume 4 Good manufacturing practice (GMP) Guidelines, Part I - Basic Requirements for Medicinal Products, Chapter 4 – Documentation. ICH E6 GCP (2) 5.5.3(f). ICH Q7 5.48. 21 CFR 58.33; .190(d); .35; .195 Specific records retention requirements are found in applicable predicate rule. For example, 21 CFR 211.180(c), (d), 108.25(g), and 108.35(h), and 58.195. 812.140(a) and (b). WHO - Technical Report Series, No. 937, 2006. Annex 4. Appendix 5, Sections 5 and 7.2.2. 21 CFR 123.9(f) GAMP Appendix O9 and O11. ISO 13485 6.2; 6.2.1; 6.2.2; 7.5 Japan CSV Guideline (Guideline on Management of Computerized Systems for Marketing Authorization Holder and Manufacturing of Drugs and Quasi-drugs, October 2010), Section 6.3.

	References				
	Old Annex 11	**211**	**820**	**11**	**Others/Guidelines**
7.2 Regular back-ups of all relevant data should be done. Integrity and accuracy of back-up data and the ability to restore the data should be checked during validation and monitored periodically.[21]					Japan's Pharmaceutical and Food Safety Bureau "Using electromagnetic records and electronic signatures for application for approval or licensing of drugs", Section 3, April 2005. Thailand CSV GMPs, Clause 517, 522, 523. Health Canada API, C.02.05, Interpretation #16. Article 19 draft Annex 2 CFDA GMP. OECD Guidance, Section 3.2, 3.11. GAMP 5, Section 4.3.6.1. ISO 27000, Section 10.5 Brasil API (RDC Resolution #69 Chapter VI Section VI Article 269) WHO Technical Report 986 Annex 2 (Section 15.9) ITIL, Service Design (Chapter 5.2.11) US FDA Data Integrity (Draft) Guidance III.1.e 211.68(b); 211.188; 211.194. Part II - Basic Requirements for Active Substances used as Starting Materials, Section 5.48. Sections 6.16 and 6.17.2, MHRA March 2018. Section 9.7, PIC/S PI 041-1 (Draft3). OMLC 7.3 and 7.4 Sections 8.2.3 and 9.8.4 Russian Federation DI Guideline Sections 12.23, 12.12.24, and 11.27, WHO QAS19_819 Health Canada GMP Guidelines 4-7. DI OECD Section 7.21

[21] Annex 11-7 is another fundamental section related with erecs integrity.

Regulatory Analysis: (Continued)

	References				
	Old Annex 11	211	820	11	Others/Guidelines
8. Printouts. 8.1 It should be possible to obtain clear printed copies of electronically stored e-records. 8.2 For records supporting batch release it should be possible to generate printouts indicating if any of the e-record has been changed since the original entry.[22] (Data quality element: Original)	11-12	211.180(c). 211.194(a).	43 FR 31508, July 21, 1978 803.1 803.10 803.14 806.30 820.40 820.180 806.1	11.10(b)	812.150, 58.15 Directive 1999/93/EC of the European Parliament and of the Council of 13 December 1999 on a Community framework for electronic signatures. PIC/S PI 011-3. FDA, Guidance for Industry Part 11, Electronic Records; Electronic Signatures — Scope and Application, August 2003. The APV Guideline, "Computerized Systems" based on Annex 11 of the EU-GMP Guideline. US FDA CPG Sec. 130.400 Use of Microfiche and/or Microfilm for Method of Records Retention. ISO 13485 4.2.3; 4.2.4. Thailand CSV GMPs, Clause 521. OECD Guidance Document, Section 3.3. Section 6.19, MHRA March 2018.

[22] Annex 11-8 is another fundamental section related with erecs integrity.

	References				
	Old Annex 11	211	820	11	Others/Guidelines
9. Audit Trails. Consideration should be given, based on a risk assessment, to building into the system the creation of a record of all GMP- relevant changes and deletions (a system generated "audit trail"). For change or deletion of GMP-relevant data the reason should be documented. Audit trails need to be available and convertible to a generally intelligible form and regularly reviewed.[23] (Data quality elements: Legible and Original)	11-10	211.180(e)	803.18 820.40	11.10(e); 11.10(k)(2); 11.50 (a)(2)	1978 US CGMP rev. Comment paragraph 186. FDA, Guidance for Industry Part 11, Electronic Records; Electronic Signatures - Scope and Application, August 2003. The APV Guideline "Computerized Systems" based on Annex 11 of the EU-GMP Guideline. PIC/S PI 011-3. PIC/S PI 041-1 (Draft3), Section 9.4 ICH Q7 Good Manufacturing Practice Guidance for Active Pharmaceutical Ingredients. ICH E6 GCP (R2) 4.9.0, 5.5.3(c), 5.5.4 21 CFR 58.130(d); 211.160(a); 211.194; 212.110(b) Glossary of the Note for Guidance on Good Clinical Practice (CPMP/ICH/135/95). ISO 13485 4.2.3 Thailand CSV GMPs, Clause 519. Health Canada API, C.02.05, Interpretation #15. OECD Guidance Document, Section 3.4. WHO Technical Report 986 Annex 2 (Section 15.9) US FDA Data Integrity (Draft) Guidance III.1.c; 7 & 8. Part II - Basic Requirements for Active Substances used as Starting Materials, Section 5.43. EU Directives 2017/1572, Article 9 Section 2. Section 6.13, MHRA March 2018.

[23] Annex 11-9 is another fundamental section related with erecs integrity.

Regulatory Analysis: (Continued)

	References				
	Old Annex 11	**211**	**820**	**11**	**Others/Guidelines**
9. Audit Trails. *Note:* In addition to the system generated audit trail, some implementation included the documentation that allows reconstruction of the course of events. Implicitly, this approach does not require a computer system generated audit trail.					Sections 8.3.1 and 8.3.2 Russian Federation DI Guideline Sections 12.14 - 12.17, WHO QAS19_819 PIC/S PI 041-1 (Draft3), Section 9.5-2. DI OECD Section 7.16
10. Change and Configuration Management Any changes to a computerised system including system configurations should only be made in a controlled manner in accordance with a defined procedure.	11-11	211.68. 211.180(e).	820.30(i). 820.70(i). 820.40.	11.10(d); 11.10(e)	ISO 90003, 2004, Sections 7.3.7 and 7.5.3.2 PIC/S PI 011-3. The APV Guideline "Computerized Systems" based on Annex 11 of the EU-GMP Guideline. WHO - Technical Report Series, No. 937, 2006. Annex 4. Section 12 Pressman, Roger S., *Software Engineering – A Practitioner's Approach*, McGraw Hill. GAMP 5 –Management Appendix M3; GAMP 5 –Operational Appendices O6 and O7. GAMP 5 Section 4.3.4.1. ISO 13485 7.3.7; 7.5.2; 4.2.3

	References				
	Old Annex 11	**211**	**820**	**11**	**Others/Guidelines**
10. Change and Configuration Management (Data quality elements: Legible and Accurate)					
11. Periodic evaluation Computerised systems should be periodically evaluated to confirm that they remain in a valid state and are compliant with GMP. Such evaluations should include, where appropriate, the current range of functionality, deviation records, incidents, problems, upgrade history, performance, reliability, ***security*** and validation status report(s). (Data quality element: Accurate)		211.68; 211.180(e).	820.20(c).	11.10(k); 11.300(b) and (e).	US FDA CPG 7132a.07, Computerized Drug Processing; Input/output Checking. ICH Q7, 12.60 WHO - Technical Report Series, No. 937, 2006. Annex 4. Appendix 5, Section 1.5 GAMP 5 Section 4.3.5. GAMP 5 –Management Appendix M3; GAMP 5 –Operational Appendices O3 and O8 58.35; 58.190; 58.195. Annex 15 clauses 23 and 45. ISO 13485 5.6; 5.6.1; 5.6.2; 5.6.3; 8.2.2; 8.5; 8.5.1. China GMPs Section 8. OECD Guidance Document, Section 3.6. ITIL, Service Design (Chapter 5.2.13) Sections 3.5 and 6.15, MHRA March 2018. Section 9.8.8 Russian Federation DI Guideline Section 4.6 in WHO QAS19_819.

Regulatory Analysis: (Continued)

	References				
	Old Annex 11	211	820	11	Others/Guidelines
12. Security 12.1 Physical and/or logical controls should be in place to restrict access to computerised system to authorised persons. Suitable methods of preventing unauthorised entry to the system may include the use of keys, pass cards, personal codes with passwords, biometrics, restricted access to computer equipment and data storage areas. 12.2 The extent of security controls depends on the criticality of the computerised system.	11-8	211.68(b) 211.160(a)		11.10(b); 11.10(c); 11.10(d); 11.10(g); 11.300.	PIC/S PI 011-3, Sections 19.2; 19.3. PIC/S PI 041-1 (Draft3), Section 9.3. ICH E6 GCP (R2) 5.5.3 (d), (e) ICH Q7 Section 5.43. 21 CFR Part 58.51; 58.190(d); 211.68(b) WHO - Technical Report Series, No. 937, 2006. Annex 4. Appendix 5 Section 4 GAMP 5, Section 4.3.7.1 GAMP 5 –Management Appendix M9; GAMP 5 –Operational Appendix O11. Japan CSV Guideline (Guideline on Management of Computerized Systems for Marketing Authorization Holder and Manufacturing of Drugs and Quasi-drugs, October 2010), Section 6.4. Thailand CSV GMPs, Clause 517. Health Canada API, C.02.05, Interpretation #15. Articles 14, 16 draft Annex 2 CFDA GMP. OECD Guidance Document, Section 3.7. ANMAT (Argentina) 5.24. ISO-27000, Sections 12.1 and 11.2. WHO Technical Report 986 Annex 2 (Section 15.9) ITIL, Service Design (Chapter 5.2.13) EU Directives 2017/1572, Article 9 Section 2.

	References				
	Old Annex 11	**211**	**820**	**11**	**Others/Guidelines**
12. Security 12.3 Creation, change, and cancellation of access authorisations should be recorded. 12.4 Management systems for data and for documents should be designed to record the identity of operators entering, changing, confirming or deleting data including date and time.[24] (Data quality elements: Attributable (12.4) and Contemporaneous (12.4))					US FDA Data Integrity (Draft) Guidance III.4 & .5. Part II - Basic Requirements for Active Substances used as Starting Materials, Section 5.43. Section 6.20, MHRA March 2018. NSF 363-14 Section 6.3.2.3 (b) OMCL Section 7.1 Sections 8.2 and 9.8.1 Russian Federation DI Guideline Sections 12.7- 12.10, WHO QAS19_819

[24] Annex 11-12 is another fundamental section related with erecs integrity.

Regulatory Analysis: (Continued)

	References				
	Old Annex 11	**211**	**820**	**11**	**Others/Guidelines**
13. Incident Management. All incidents, not only system failures and data errors, should be reported and assessed. The root cause of a critical incident should be identified and should form the basis of corrective and preventive actions.	11-17	211.100(b)	820.100		ICH Q7A Good Manufacturing Practice Guidance for Active Pharmaceutical Ingredients, Section 5.46. ICH E6, Section 5.1.3. GAMP 5 - Operational Appendices O4. O5,and O7. ISO 13485 8.5; 8.5.1; 8.5.2; 8.5.3 Japan CSV Guideline (Guideline on Management of Computerized Systems for Marketing Authorization Holder and Manufacturing of Drugs and Quasi-drugs, October 2010), Sections 6.7 and 7.2. China GMPs, Sections 5 and 6. Thailand CSV GMPs, Clause 526. Health Canada API, C.02.015 Interpretation #19. Articles 20 and 21 draft Annex 2 CFDA GMP. OECD Guidance Document, Section 3.8. ANMAT (Argentina) 5.27. US FDA General Principles of Software Validation, Section 5.2.7. Part II - Basic Requirements for Active Substances used as Starting Materials, Section 5.46. Section 3.9, MHRA March 2018

	References				
	Old Annex 11	211	820	11	Others/Guidelines
14. Electronic Signature. Electronic records may be signed electronically. Electronic signatures are expected to: have the same impact as hand-written signatures within the boundaries of the company[25], be permanently linked to their respective record, include the time and date that they were applied. (Data quality element: Contemporaneous)				11.3(b)(7); 11.10(e); 11.50; .70, .100, .200, .300	EU GMP Chapter 4 Principle Annex 11-8.1, 9, 12.4, 17 ICH Q7A Good Manufacturing Practice Guidance for Active Pharmaceutical Ingredients, Section 5.43. Electronic Signatures in Global and National Commerce (E-Sign), a US federal law. (available at: http://thomas.loc.gov/cgi-bin/query/z?c106:S.761:) 21 CFR 58.33; .81; .35; .120; .185 Japan's Pharmaceutical and Food Safety Bureau "Using electromagnetic records and electronic signatures for application for approval or licensing of drugs", Section 4, April 2005. Article 22 draft Annex 2 CFDA GMP. Guidance Document, Section 3.10. US FDA Data Integrity (Draft) Guidance III.11 Section 6.14, MHRA March 2018. Sections 12.18 – 12.19, WHO QAS19_819 DI OECD Section 7.17

[25] The phase "within the boundaries of the company" clarifies that such signatures applied to records maintained by the regulated company are not subject to Directive 1999/93/EC on a Company framework for esigs, nor the 2000/31/EC Directive on electronic commerce, nor any associated national regulations of EU member states on such topics.

Regulatory Analysis: (Continued)

	References				
	Old Annex 11	**211**	**820**	**11**	**Others/Guidelines**
15. Batch release. When a computerized system is used for recording certification and batch release, the system should allow only Qualified Persons to certify the release of the batches and it should clearly identify and record the person releasing or certifying the batches. This should be performed using an electronic signature. (Data quality element: Attributable)	11-19	211.68 211.186 211.192 211.188(b)(11) 211.188(a)		11.70; Sub Part C	21 CFR 211.68 The APV Guideline "Computerized Systems" based on Annex 11 of the EU-GMP Guideline. 11-9; 11-14 EC Directive 2001/83. Thailand CSV GMPs, Clause 528. Article 21 draft Annex 2 CFDA GMP.

	References				
	Old Annex 11	211	820	11	Others/Guidelines
16. Business Continuity. For the availability of computerised systems supporting critical processes, provisions should be made to ensure continuity of support for those processes in the event of a system breakdown (e.g., a manual or alternative system). The time required to bring the alternative arrangements into use should be based on risk and appropriate for a particular system and the business process it supports. These arrangements should be adequately documented and tested.[26]	11-15 11-16				PIC/S PI 011-3. GAMP 5, Sections 4.3.6.2 and 4.3.6.3. GAMP 5 –Operational Appendix O10. Thailand CSV GMPs, Clause 524, 525. OECD Guidance Document, Section 3.12. ANMAT (Argentina) 5.29. ICH Q7, Section 5.48. NSF 363-14 Section 6.3.2.3 (d) 2001/83, Article 81. Section 6.20, MHRA March 2018. Section 9.6.6 Russian Federation DI Guideline

[26] Annex 11-16 is another fundamental section related with erecs integrity.

Regulatory Analysis: (Continued)

	References				
	Old Annex 11	**211**	**820**	**11**	**Others/Guidelines**
17. Archiving. Data may be archived. This data should be checked for accessibility, readability and integrity. If relevant changes are to be made to the system (e.g., computer equipment or programs), then the ability to retrieve the data should be ensured and tested. **(Data integrity element: Legible)**		211.68(b). 211.180(e).		11.10(c)	Scientific Archivists Group, A Guide to Archiving of Electronic Records, 2014 www.sagroup.org.uk/images/documents/AGuidetoArchivingElectronicRecordsv1.pdf DOD 5015.2-STD, Design Criteria Standard for E-records Management Software Applications. GAMP 5 –Operational Appendix O13. GAMP GPG: Electronic Data Archiving, 2007. Draft OECD Guidance Document, Section 3.12. Scientific Archivists Group, "A Guide to Archiving of Electronic Records" ITIL, Service Design (Chapter 5.2.13) Sections 6.17.1, MHRA March 2018. EU Directives 2017/1572, Article 9 Section 2. OMCL Section 6.9 and 7.4 Section 8.4.2and 9.8.7 Russia Federation DI Guideline. Section 9.7, PIC/S PI 041-1 (Draft3) DI OECD Section 7.22.

Revision History

Date	Update Reason
02-Feb-2011	Creation of the Annex 11 matrix.
21-Feb-2011	Updated format of matrix and updated based on various references.
08-Mar-2011	Updated various 21 CFR 820 references based on the US FDA General Principles of Software Validation, January 2002, CDRH and CBER.
13-Mar-2011	Updated various 21 CFR 211 references based on the US FDA Guide to Inspection of Computerized Systems in Drug Processing, February 1983.
22-Mar-2011	Updated various 21 CFR 11 references based on regulation. Add raw data references. Updated periodic review based on comments by Jeffrey Torres.
31-Mar-2011	Updated "Principle" reference based on US FDA CPG 7348.810 - Sponsors, CROs, and Monitors. Updated various 21 CFR 820 references based on another matrix correlating various regulatory requirements. Updated various references based on ICH E6 GCP, 21 CFR 58, and 21 CFR 312.
09-Apr-2011	Added ISO 14971 as a reference. Updated 11-7 based on 21 CFR 820.
23-Apr-2011	Updated various references based on various CFRs.
11-May-2011	Updated based on regulations for Computerized Systems Used in Medical Device Clinical Investigations, 21 CFR 812.
12-Jun-2011	Added 211.194(d) in Data Section; Added reference on my recent article on Requirements Management, published by IVT; Section 4, added the Blood Establishment Computer System Validation in the User's Facility, October 2007 (Draft Guidance); added as a reference EMA/INS/GCP/454280/2010 GCP Inspectors Working Group (GCP IWG), "*Reflection paper on expectations for electronic source data and data transcribed to electronic data collection tools in clinical trials.*"; Updated various references based on 21 CFR 58.
03-Aug-2011	Added regulatory requirements about 820 based on the US FDA Medical Devices QS Manual: A small entity compliance guide, Chapter 7; added in periodic review reference of ICH Q7, 12.6; Modifications to Old-New Annex 11 mappings.
23-Aug-2011	Added WHO Technical Report Series, No. 937, 2006. Annex 4. Appendix 5. 2006
26-Aug-2011	Added Electronic Signatures in Global and National Commerce (E-Sign), a US federal law

Regulatory Analysis: (Continued)

Date	Update Reason
25-Sep-2011	Added GAMP 5 Cross references (Yves Samson); added definition of Test Methods based APV guideline.
24-Oct-11	Added Tissues Reg 21 CFR 1271.160(d); Food 21 CFR 123.9(f)
17-Mar-2012	Updated based on NEMA Presentation. “Part 11 Recommendations for Changes”, June 2004.
21-Oct-12	Updated based on presentation FDA Public Meeting June 2004 (R. Eaton and R. Nabar)
15-Nov-2012	Updated various references-based ICH Q10, ISPE GAMP COP Annex 11 – Interpretation, July/August 2011.
2-Dec-12	Updated based on Brazilian GMPs, Title VII Resolution of the Executive Board No. 17, Computerized Information Systems. This can be found on page 109 de 148, http://www.in.gov.br/imprensa/visualiza/index.jsp?jornal=1&pagina=94&data=19/04/2010
07-Apr-13	Updated guideline Blood Establishment Computer System Validation in the User’s Facility, from October 2007 (Draft Guidance) to April 2013 (Final Guidance).
24-Aug-13	Updated with ISO 134854.
24-Oct-13	Added Japanese CSV Guidelines (Guidelines on Management of Computerized Systems for Marketing Authorization Holders and Manufacturers of Drugs and Quasi-drugs, October 2010) and Japan’s Pharmaceutical and Food Safety Bureau “Using electromagnetic records and electronic signatures for application for approval or licensing of drugs”, April 2005.
31-Oct-13	Added State Food and Drug Administration, P.R. China, March 2011 and Thailand CSV GMPs contained in the Prescription of Details regarding and Procedures of Manufacture of Modern Medicinal Products in compliance with Drug Lawa B.E.2554.
08-Feb-14	Added 91/412/EEC; WHO, Technical Report Series No. 981 PDA, Technical Report No. 32; CEFIC CSV Guide Rev 2, December 2002. Health Canada GMP Guidelines for API (GUI-0104) Dec 2013.
08-Feb-14b	Corrected copy. Added couple of sections left out from the Health Canada GMP Guidelines for API.
26-Mar-14	Updated application sections based on ICH E6 GCP.
09-Jul-14	Incorrect references in 21 CFR Part 58, Security. China Food & Drug Administration (CFDA) draft of GMP Annex 2 Computerized Systems.

Date	Update Reason
12-Sep-14	Added reference GAMP GPG: Electronic Data Archiving, 2007 to Archiving; Added reference GAMP GPG: IT Infrastructure Control and Compliance, 2005 to Principle b. Added reference ISO/TR 14969:2004 Medical devices – Quality management systems – Guidance on the application of ISO 13485. Added EudraLex, The Rules Governing Medicinal Products in the European Union Volume 4, Good Manufacturing Practice, Medicinal Products for Human and Veterinary Use, Chapter 7: Outsourced Activities, January 2013 to Suppliers and Service Providers.
23-Sep-14	Added Draft OECD Guidance Document – The Application of GLP Principles to Computerised Systems, September 2014. (Note: The entries related with this DRAFT, were replaced with the final document. Refer 21Feb18 entry.)
10-Oct-14	Based on the definition by the NIST (SP 800-33), highlighted the data integrity related items on Annex 11.
19-Dec-14	Added ISO 90003:2014 applicable sections related with Configuration Management and applicable development phase activities.
05-Mar-15	Added ICH E6, Guideline for GCP (Jun 1996). Added Administracion Nacional de Medicamentos, Alimentos y Tecnologia Medicas (ANMAT) (Argentina's Ministerio de Salud Presidencia de la Nacion). Added ISO/IEC 27000 Information Security Management Systems. Added US FDA General Principles of Software Validation. Fixed minor errors.
01-Aug-15	In 11-17 added Scientific Archivists Group, "A Guide to Archiving of Electronic Records", as a reference. Added Brazil API Regulations (RDC Resolution #69)
14-Nov-15	Added WHO Guide regarding the Principles of GMP Technical Report 986, Annex 2 WHO good manufacturing practices for pharmaceutical products: main principles. Added ITIL Service Design, Chapter 5.2 – Management of data and information, 2011 Edition
22-Apr-16	Added US FDA Guidance for Industry: Data Integrity and Compliance with CGMP (Draft)
11-Aug-16	Added Part II - Basic Requirements for Active Substances used as Starting Materials Added EMA Q&A: GMP Data Integrity, August 2016. Added MHRA GxP Data Integrity Definitions and Guidance for Industry, July 2016 (Draft) Added PIC/S, Good Practices for Data Management and Integrity in Regulated GMP/GCP Environments," PI 041-1 (Draft2), August 2016. TGA intends to reference the PIC/S Good Practices for Data Management and Integrity in Regulated GMP/GDP Environments, PI 041-1 (Draft 2) Added WHO Guidance on Good Data and Record Management Practices, Technical Report 966, Annex 5 WHO Expert Committee on Specifications for Pharmaceutical Preparations.
28-Sep-16	Added NSF/IPEC/ANSI 363 – 2014 Good Manufacturing Practices (GMP) for Pharmaceutical Excipients

Regulatory Analysis: (Continued)

Date	Update Reason
24-Sep-17	ICH E6 (R2) GCP Guideline (2016); Updated articles in EU GMP Directive 2003/94/EC with applicable articles in the new Directive 2017/1572; OMCL Management of Documents and Records (January 2016).
04-Nov-17	Integration of Q13 in Added EMA Q&A: GMP Data Integrity, August 2016 with Added US FDA Guidance for Industry: Data Integrity and Compliance with CGMP (Draft).
21-Feb-18	Replaced "Data integrity element" with "Data quality element": Replaced Draft OECD Guidance Document – The Application of GLP Principles to Computerised Systems, September 2014 with the final version April 2016.
04-Apr-18	The entries related with MHRA GxP Data Integrity Definitions and Guidance for Industry, July 2016 (Draft) were replaced with the final document. Refer 11Aug16 entry. The final guidance document, MHRA GxP Data Integrity Guidance and Definitions was published on March 2018.
26-May-19	Updated entries with Russia Federal State Institute of Drugs and Good Practices (Draft) https://drive.google.com/file/d/1lMdc7QQkz6h_tinHpJBvb-WMby6WNe4C/view?usp=sharing
03-Nov-19	Entries updated based on WHO QAS19_819_data_integrity (Draft October 2019) and CEFIC Data Integrity Best Practices Guide for API (FINAL March 2019). Updated PIC/S PI Draft 2 references with PIC/S 041_1 Draft_3_Guidance on Data Integrity.
23-Feb-20	Updated based on Health Canada, Good Manufacturing Practices (GMP) Guidelines - 2018 Edition, Version 3 (GUI-0001). Updated using data integrity elements only in Canadian Guideline.
30-Mar-20	Correlated 211.68(a) and EU Annex-11 Principle 1.
29-Jul-20	Updated based on Guide to CSV, Anvisa (April 2020)
09-Sep-20	OECD_Advisory_Document_on_GLP_Data_Integrity (Draft 20200807); NMPA (former CFDA), Data Record and Management (December 2020)

INDEX

A

C

D

E

Q

R

S

T

U

V

W

X

Y